DEDICATED TO MY PARENTS

This book is dedicated to my parents.

Words can't express how grateful I am to you both for always supporting me in life. Everything I have achieved would not be possible if it wasn't for you both, and the unconditional love and support you have provided me.

Thank you for always being there by my side when my crohn's disease landed me in hospital, in A&E and providing me with comfort and a safe environment to recover in when I needed it the most.

Thank you both for teaching me the value of working hard and honestly to not only achieve my dreams but to help others and positively contribute to society.

May God bless you both.

REVIEWS

"Whether you're a clinician or have recently been diagnosed with IBD, this honest and authentic account, will provide helpful and informative insight of the reality of living with IBD. This well researched, easy to read, evidenced based handbook, tackles the many questions newly diagnosed patients need the answers to, whilst managing to dispel the numerous myths surrounding IBD and sharing the facts you need to know about living with the disease.

Ziyad talks candidly about his personal experience including the reality of how seriously life can be impacted and the complexity of developing disordered eating. This book highlights the challenges and reality of living with this often life changing and debilitating disease and touches on the rarely discussed social impact of navigating life, work and relationships with the disease.

~ This handbook is a must read for anyone living with IBD."

Hala El-Shafie, *Bariatric surgery and Eating Disorders Specialist Registered Dietitian*

"Ziyad has put together an incredibly comprehensive book covering everything from how the gut works, the basics of inflammatory bowel disease (IBD) to the importance of good nutrition for those with IBD.

Having followed Ziyad's Instagram page, **The Grumbling Gut**, for several years now and knowing that he has experienced the struggles of IBD first hand, I can't think of a better person to have put together such a thorough guide. This is an invaluable resource for anyone with IBD, as well as for those wishing to learn more about this group of conditions and how they can help people with it. Huge Congrats on such a unique and fantastic book!"

Dr Michelle Braude, *MBBS, BSc Nutrition, author of The Food Effect Diet and The Food Effect Diet Vegan*

THE GRUMBLING GUT

TABLE OF
CONTENTS

FOREWARD

Hello, and welcome! My name is Ziyad, and I am the creator, founder and person behind **The Grumbling Gut.**

As a qualified NHS research radiographer, nutrition and weight management advisor and crohn's disease patient this book combines my area of interest and expertise to offer you a full, easy to understand nutrition guide specifically for inflammatory bowel disease (IBD).

This book isn't your regular 'diet' or 'gut health' recipe book that are swamping the market at the moment, as it has been designed to debunk the myths about IBD and nutrition by providing you with the latest evidenced-based information.

This book is different as I want it to be able to:
- Share my struggle with crohn's disease
- Teach you the basics of IBD & nutrition
- Allow you to understand why IBD causes nutritional deficiencies
- Provide you with tips that make living with IBD easier
- Help to encourage you to see that food is not the enemy when it comes to IBD

I created **The Grumbling Gut** as a blog in 2017 to raise awareness of IBD, and I hope this book can contribute to that. I want to be able to encourage and inspire others to speak up about their illnesses to help beat the stigma and show that not every disability is visible.

BEFORE WE BEGIN...

Medical terms are highlighted in **bold** and are explained in the glossary. Recommendations relating to IBD, general health, IBD tips, signs/symptoms which require immediate medical attention, IBD myths other useful bits of information will be displayed in text boxes throughout this book.

So, let's get started and I hope you enjoy this book!

ZIYAD AL-DIBOUNI

ZIYAD AL-DIBOUNI (BSc,MSc)
@thegrumblinggut

CHAPTER 1: INTRODUCTION
YOU DON'T LOOK SICK

For the first sixteen years of my life, I had a very good relationship with food. Put anything in front of me and it would be gone in a few seconds. However, shortly after my GCSE's that began to change when I was diagnosed with one of the two main forms of inflammatory bowel disease (IBD), crohn's disease, an incurable illness. Even though I am in remission now it didn't happen overnight but took many years of trying different medications and multiple surgeries to get to that stage. You'd never be able to tell that I have crohn's disease just by looking at me (that's the whole point of an invisible illness) and often or not I hear the many variations of the phrase "you don't look sick to me" when I tell people about my illness.

I can't pinpoint the exact moment I started to experience symptoms as they gradually occurred and it was very easy to pass off any irregularity in my health to just being stressed out by exams. I won't bore you with the nitty gritty details but the timeline from when I experienced symptoms to getting my diagnosis was just over one year. Throughout that year there were numerous trips to A&E and my local GP, but I was repeatedly told by every doctor I saw that my symptoms were due to exam stress and a lack of fibre in my diet. I felt like I was being a burden to my doctors and wasting their time and that it got to the point where I was seriously contemplating the possibility that everything I was going through might all just be in my head and that there was nothing wrong with me, especially when my blood tests kept coming back as normal.

Looking back now it is easy to see why I could never get a definitive diagnosis or even a referral to a specialist as aside from stomach cramps and going to the toilet a little more often than usual I wasn't displaying any of the more severe symptoms of crohn's disease. I remember waking up one morning in so much pain that I couldn't go to school and ended up having to take some time off. That morning was the first time I notice blood after going to the toilet and it seriously freaked me out! I was so shocked and so embarrassed that I didn't tell anyone hoping that everything would resolve on its own and eventually go away. The thing is when you have IBD you can feel so rough yet somehow you still manage to go about your day-to-day activities and even though I didn't know I had crohn's disease, that is exactly what I did after gaining back some strength. I went back to school, I studied, went out with my friends, attended my football training sessions and matches for both my school and club. For me, life just went on and I accepted whatever I went through as part of my normal routine, where I'd have to take some time off school because I would be unwell.

Although I had accepted this as part of my life, the severity and frequency of my symptoms started to increase to the point where I would be up all night going to the toilet, losing a lot of blood, not getting much sleep and sometimes feeling so nauseated that I'd actually be sick. It was like some cruel joke. Be in pain, vomit, bleed and repeat. Trying to live a normal life and keep up appearances was hard enough but I was getting increasingly more tired, fatigued and sicker, missing a lot of school to the point where my friends and teachers started to notice. I feel I could have got away with it despite it being a regular occurrence but it was the drastic change in my physical appearance due to extreme weight loss that gave it away and the reason why people would ask a lot of questions. I would always just brush off any comments about my appearance or my health as I never really knew how to answer mainly because I didn't know what was going on with me. I was always healthy and I don't drink or smoke to me I always believed that this was just how life was going to be from now on and that things will get better and go back to normal soon and all I had to do was be patient.

How very wrong I was. It wasn't until my relationship with food changed drastically, where things started to get worse because what little weight I had on me soon disappeared. It was at this point where I really did start to doubt that exam stress and the 'lack of fibre' in my diet could really do this to my body and that what I was going through was very real and certainly wasn't just in my head.

"

YOU DON'T LOOK SICK TO ME!

... _____

My Unknown Eating Disorder

Looking back at what I went through it is clear to see that experiencing symptoms of crohn's disease did cause me to develop an eating disorder without me even realising it. Eating disorders are complex mental illnesses which can occur in anyone causing them to have an unhealthy attitude towards food (which can involve either eating too much or too little and becoming obsessed with your weight and body shape) causing ill health.

So where does crohn's disease fit into all of this?

I will mention more about the causes of IBD in this book but to summarise quickly no one knows exactly what causes it with current theories being revolved around having a western diet being a potential contributing factor among other things. If you haven't guessed it from my name alone, I have Arabic heritage and, in my culture, (and many other cultures) food plays a massive role and I have been fortunate enough to be brought up on wholesome, nutritious homecooked meals made from natural ingredients.

However, I was born and raised in the UK so naturally a western diet was adopted and I'll be the first to admit that home-cooked meals didn't make up my entire diet as I was partial to the odd take away now and then. It's because of this that it never made sense to me why doctors would think that I lacked fibre in my diet when for the most part I was eating healthy and nutritious foods on a daily basis.

During the year I spent undiagnosed, I noticed one common thing every time I experienced symptoms and that was, they would always start a few hours after eating something. It didn't matter what I ate but especially after dinner, I would start my night time routine of being in pain, vomiting and bleeding while trying to fit in a few moments of sleep. Food should taste good and it is meant to nurture your body and making this subconscious connection of 'eating means being in pain', I started to become fussy about what I ate and in no time at all my perception of food changed from friend to foe. I developed such a negative and unhealthy relationship with food and I started to fear it and like any other sixteen-year-old who has all the answers I decided to take matters in my own hands.

Using my infinite wisdom and medical experience available to me at that age I decided the best remedy to not being in pain was not to eat. I know. Not the smartest thing I ever did. I didn't go off food completely but my habits and attitude towards food changed drastically as I started to limit the amount of food I would eat, become less adventurous about food, obsess about the ingredients and in some cases avoid food completely.

The type of eating disorder I developed because of my crohn's disease is known as: **Avoidant/Restrictive Food Intake Disorder (ARFID)** and it is a type of eating disorder where people either avoid certain types of food or limit the amount they eat. At the time I would have never considered that I had an eating disorder and it was only recently where I felt comfortable enough to not only admit it to myself but speak about it publicly.

There are many reasons why people can develop ARFID and in my case I associated my night-time routine of pain, vomit, bleed repeat to be caused by food which lead me to develop feelings of fear and anxiety about eating. It is important to say that this was my version of ARFID and although I am sure many can relate to what I went through, everyone's ARFID or relationship around food and their reasons for going through it is different.

Needless to say, having ARFIDand eating what I considered my 'safe foods' did not do my body any favours and only accelerated the rate of weight loss and frequency of my symptoms.

Throughout this time my family noticed my unusual behaviour and obsession around food and were starting to get concerned about my health and despite my constant reassurances to them that I'm fine, my physical appearance said otherwise. I remember being taken to the doctors by my parents and due to their insistence that something wasn't right, the drastic change in my physical appearance and my recent symptoms of stomach pains and bleeding was all it took for my doctors to start taking me seriously.

A referral to a specialist was made, after a blood test showed I was very anaemic, had raised inflammatory markers and in general was in really poor health, where I eventually got my diagnosis.

BEHAVIOURAL & PHYSICAL SIGNS OF AN EATING DISORDER

IF YOU NOTICE THESE SIGNS IN YOURSELF OR SOMEONE ELSE SEEK MEDICAL ATTENTION FROM YOUR DOCTOR OR AN EATING DISORDER CHARITY HELPLINE

- Making yourself sick on purpose after eating a meal
- Mood swings/changes in normal behaviour
- Eating food very quickly
- Lying about the amount of food you've eaten
- Becoming obsessed with weight and body shape
- Starting to have problems with digestion
- Start to become obsessive about exercising
- Feeling cold, tired and light headed all the time
- Having strict routines and habits around food
- Not getting a period (women only)
- Wearing loose/baggy clothing to hide physical appearance
- Eating very little food
- Dramatic weight loss
- Avoiding social scenarios when food is involved

The Diagnosis

Before eventually getting my diagnosis, I had every investigation under the sun. I had x-rays, barium swallows, MRI scans and colonoscopies all of which I was experiencing for the first time. This was also my first major experience of being a patient and in some romanticised way gave me an insight into my future career as a diagnostic radiographer.

I still remember the consultation I had and being told that there was no cure for crohn's disease and it really felt like the proverbial rug had been pulled out from underneath me. There were so many things going through my head and I experienced such a mixture of emotions. I felt relieved that not only did I finally have an answer to what was causing my health to decline and that it confirmed this wasn't all in my head like I was left to believe. But on the other hand, there was a lot of fear, anxiety and uncertainty of what my future would actually hold for me and it felt like some cruel joke was being played on me yet again as up until all this I was your 'normal' healthy person.

The normality of life that I was so accustomed to before becoming ill had changed drastically already and things kept on changing again once I began treatment. I didn't really have much confidence in the doctors that were treating me either and I saw many different specialists as it really did feel their treatment plan was "let's throw what we've got against the wall and see what sticks". It felt more like trial and error than a thought-out plan and most of the medications I was initially on had so many side effects that were almost as bad as the initial symptoms of crohn's disease itself. I literally felt dehumanised and like I was being seen as a set of symptoms on a checklist after each appointment and it was never really explained to me or taken into consideration as to how these medications would impact my daily life. I always had so much respect for doctors and the medical community, especially as I wanted a career in the medical field, but I was slowing losing faith in the whole healthcare system.

Fortunately, after one more change in specialist my faith was restored as the specialist that I see till this day not only listened to my opinions but explained everything that he had planned for my treatment plan and without him I would not be in remission.

"

EVEN THOUGH I AM IN
REMISSION NOW IT
DIDN'T HAPPEN
OVERNIGHT BUT TOOK
MANY YEARS OF TRYING
DIFFERENT
MEDICATIONS AND
MULTIPLE SURGERIES
TO GET TO THAT STAGE.

"

The Fight with Food

Even though I was starting to feel better due to new medications I still had a very bad attitude towards food and so I was referred to a dietician. I feel this was the turning point for me in not only repairing my relationship with food but also putting me in the right direction to trying to gain some weight back.

Anyone with IBD who has lost weight can tell you it is the hardest thing to try and put back on no matter how much you eat and for years my weight and the topic of food has been such an issue. The trouble was due to my ARFID and associating food with pain that my diet was very limited even though I knew now that the pain I experienced after meal times weren't necessarily due to the what I was eating, the damage was already done. I wasn't very adventurous when it came to food and instead of eating the wholesome foods my mum would cook – and to give you some idea of timelines I just started university which even though I still lived at home – I would end up buying 'outside' or fast foods, eating them while waiting for the bus home.

This was something my dietician wanted to tackle and so I had to keep track of everything I was eating in a food diary so I could then take it back to my dietician for review. I could tell that she wasn't impressed that I was still having fast food – in my defence it was less than before - but instead of making me feel guilty about it we spoke about why I was choosing these foods and started to talk about my eating habits and what my perception of food was. I did notice that after each session I became more aware of my food choices and was slowly rediscovering that food was not the enemy and food should be celebrated and enjoyed. However, all good things must come to an end and that's what it felt like when I suffered a flare up which made me very sick and I lost whatever little weight I managed to gain and was pretty much back to square one.

After this flare up and my latest colonoscopy showing severe inflammation despite the medication I was on it was decided by my consultant that I should give my bowel a break and so I started on exclusive enteral nutrition (EEN) under the guidance of my dietician. I didn't know it at the time but this was the start of the healing process for my relationship with food and I will explain more in this book as to what EEN is and how it works. But to put it simply I was put on a liquid diet where I wasn't allowed to eat any solid foods for the duration of six weeks and aside from fluids, I could only have specially formulated drinks for sustenance.

Even though these drinks came in different flavours which didn't taste that bad, it was so hard to be around food because I wasn't allowed to have any. Meal times at home is the time where we come together as a family and sit with each other to eat but I soon found this very difficult to participate in because all I was allowed to have were my formulated drinks. You never notice how good food looks when you're all of a sudden not allowed to have it and how much of our lives actually revolve around it. It became increasingly difficult to actually socialise with my friends at university as well especially when it came to lunch time or meeting up after lectures and I would often make up excuses like I was meeting other friends or had a tutor meeting so I could go somewhere private and drink my formulated drink, just to avoid any awkward questions.

In the run up to coming off these drinks I saw my dietician often to discuss the reintroduction process of food and I was actually looking forward to it. For the first time in a long time I felt better and had a bit more energy and my overall mood and outlook on life with crohn's disease improved. The reintroduction phase was tough but worth it as I had to start off very slowly in order to get my body used to processing food again but it was all worth it as my relationship with food started to change for the better and remembering the different meals I thought looked good when I was on enteral nutrition, I started to become a bit more adventurous in what I would eat. This was the beginning of the road to recovery and the changes in me eating a wider variety of food was showing as I started to gain weight but the real hero is my mum who would make sure to cook me different foods to the rest of the family if I didn't fancy the main meal or if it had my trigger food. Thank you, mum, love you.

The Grumbling Gut - How it all started

My mission to help raise awareness and help educate people about IBD has influenced every aspect of my life. I feel my experiences as a patient has influenced the way in which I provide care for my own patients through my profession as a diagnostic radiographer. I have personally had some not so pleasant experiences in hospital and can relate to my patients because 'I've been there', but the most important thing I've realised through my own journey is the value of speaking up and having your opinions heard. Like many patients that go see their doctors I always put my trust in them and assumed they have all the answers, and while in some cases their professional opinions may be correct it is still nice to have your view listened to and respected. I have learnt that not only do I have a voice and a say as to what happens to me when being treated but I also have more control in the decision-making process than what I first realised. This is what I try toconvey to the patients that I meet when at work on a daily basis.

Yes, as a healthcare professional I have my professional opinion on what is the best course of action to take based on clinical experience but what many tend to forget is at the end of those decisions is a real person, with real feelings and opinions and not just a name on a medical form. I find it is so important to involve patients in the decision-making process allowing them to have the chance to use their voices and express their concerns and opinions and I have no doubt that encouraging them to do this will help them feel more valued and less like a checklist of symptoms as I was made to feel like during the early stages of my diagnosis.

Despite my crohn's disease being in remission the one thing that has always stayed with me was the embarrassment of having it which has always prevented me speaking about it. The decision to start talking about my personal experiences with IBD wasn't a conscious one and just sort of happened. I started to blog about my experiences with crohn's disease in 2017, anonymously at first and for some reason and I am not sure why, something compelled me to share my story in public on social media. Needless to say, many of my friends were shocked to find out that I have a chronic illness and the response was overwhelming at first. I started to get messages and comments that ranged from "what is crohn's disease" to "I had no idea you were sick" and surprisingly some messages of along the lines of "my family member or close friend has that". Reading these messages made me feel less embarrassed and wished I was more open about it from the start, but one thing was glaringly obvious from the start: more awareness was needed.

While I played around with a few different names for my blog and social media handle, I settled upon **The Grumbling Gut** (@thegrumblinggut), because what could describe IBD more perfectly than that?! With this new identity I dedicated my social media to raising awareness, providing education and support to those living with IBD in the hope to encourage and inspire others while showing the world that not every disability is visible.

CHAPTER 2: UNDERSTANDING THE GUT
GUT HEALTH

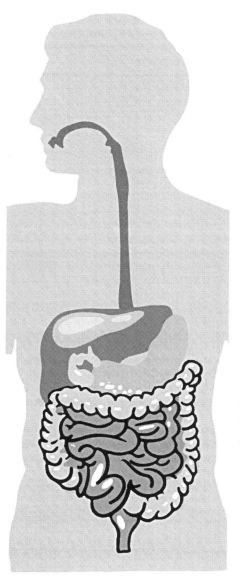

Gut health, especially now a days, is such a hot topic and there does seem to be an endless stream of advice on what to do to achieve optimal gut health. It can be so hard to separate the facts from fiction and which source to trust, especially if you have bowel conditions such as crohn's disease and ulcerative colitis.

For those that do suffer with gastrointestinal conditions, in being able to understand how the gut works, what impacts the functioning of the gut and the role of nutrition on the gut can help in gaining a better understanding of their condition and take steps to help in managing symptoms.

Before we dive right into what exactly is 'gut health', it is important to note that we are all different and there is no one size fits all when it comes to nutrition and gut health. But for now, let's take a closer look at what actually makes up the gut and the process of digestion.

What is the gut?

The digestive system is also known as the gastrointestinal tract and it is involved in digesting all the food we eat, absorbing the essential nutrients we need and turning our food into poo! Food provides us with this energy and it is digested in the body by mechanical and chemical processes.

Mechanical digestion involves the physical breakdown of food either by chewing or the physical movement within the body whereas chemical digestion requires the use of enzymes and hormones that change the composition of the food you have eaten to help break them down. This makes it easier for our body to readily absorb the essential fats, proteins, carbohydrates, vitamins and minerals we need to maintain the normal functioning of our body.

Our digestive system consists of our mouth, oesophagus, stomach, liver, pancreas, small intestine, large intestine, rectum and anus. All of these are involved in turning the food we eat into the essential components that we require to function normally in just five steps:

Step 1: Ingestion

Body parts involved: The mouth

Ingestion is simply referring to the presence of food in your mouth once you've taken a bite out of the meal you're eating. When we take a bite of food our teeth crush and grind the food which is physically breaking it into smaller pieces. This process is known as **mastication** and is a form of mechanical digestion which is assisted by the tongue that helps manipulate the food when chewing. The saliva in our mouths is secreted by the salivary glands and is a fluid that is made up of many different components including the enzymes, amylase and lipase. These enzymes start the process of chemical digestion and help break down and lubricate the food making it easier to swallow as it travels down the oesophagus.

Step 2: Propulsion

Body parts involved: The oesophagus

When you chew food, you form what is called a food bolus which is then swallowed andtravels down your oesophagus by a process called **peristalsis**, which is the name given to wave like muscle contractions which pushes the food bolus towards your stomach. The oesophagus main function is to act as a connection between your mouth and stomach facilitating the transportation of chewed food.

Step 3: Digestion

Body parts involved: Stomach, Small Intestines, Gall Bladder, Pancreas

Both mechanical and chemical digestion occur in the stomach which you can think of as a bag that holds your food. Your stomach can hold roughly 4 litres of food and liquid which are mixed with a number of gastric juices to assist in chemical digestion. This gastric juice is made up of a combination of mucus, hydrochloric acid (HCl) and enzymes that all work together to help in the process of digestion. The mucus secreted in your stomach, provides a protective coating for your stomach against the HCl that is released which helps to destroy any harmful bacteria that you may have ingested. This HCl also has another function, which is converting an enzyme called pepsinogen into its active form (pepsin) where it is then able to break down proteins within the food bolus received. One of the other components of gastric juices is a glycoprotein called intrinsic factor, which binds onto vitamin B12 making it easier to be absorbed by the body in the ileum of the small intestines, while gastric lipases helps to break down fats within the food bolus.

The hormone gastrin is released into the bloodstream as a response to your stomach stretching to accommodate the food and drink you have ingested. This hormone stimulates the release of gastric juices in your stomach as well as causing the muscles in your stomach to contract in a wave like fashion to assist in digesting your food. These continuous waves like contractions allow all the contents of your stomach to be mixed together, physically broken down and form a mixture called chyme, which is passed from the stomach into the duodenum of the small intestines.

"IT WAS LIKE SOME CRUEL JOKE:

PAIN. VOMIT. BLEED. REPEAT."

The small intestines consist of three portions: the duodenum, jejunum and ileum, and is roughly 3 metres (10 feet) in length. It is here within the small intestines where your food is also digested, and all the nutrients are absorbed into the blood stream. Bile is secreted into the duodenum, via bile ducts, to assist in the digestion of fats and vitamins, while pancreatic juices containing enzymes (trypsinogen, chymotrypsinogen and procarboxypeptidase) that are their inactive form to prevent them from breaking down the pancreas. Once these pancreatic enzymes are released into the duodenum an enzyme called enteropeptidase activates them converting trypsinogen to trypsin, chymotrypsinogen to chymotrypsin and procarboxypeptidase to carboxypeptidase which all help in breaking down proteins. Pancreatic juice also contains the enzymes amylase, lipase and nuclease, which are in their active forms, to help break down starch, fats and nucleic acids respectively.

Step 4: Absorption

Body parts involved: Small and Large Intestines

Once all the food you have eaten is broken down into its simplest forms, can the nutrients pass through the walls of the small intestines and into the bloodstream to be delivered around the body. The walls of the small intestines have microscopic finger-like projections called villi which increases its surface area. This surface area is further increased as these villi also have mini finger-like projections known as microvilli which massively increases the area of the small intestines that comes into contact with the chyme (partially digested food from your stomach). A process called **segmentation** occurs in the small intestines where muscle contractions ensures that every bit of the chyme meets the intestinal wall allowing for maximum absorption of nutrients. This segmentation also allows the chyme to be mixed with bile and pancreatic juices made by the liver and pancreas respectively.

Once the small intestines have absorbed all the available nutrients it can, what's left over is moved along into the large intestines (colon). Most people think that no absorption of nutrients occurs here as what is left is just waste products, but this is not true. The large intestines continue to break down what it received from the small intestines absorbing any water and **electrolytes** available. The colon is also home to many kinds of microbes which use these waste products as a form of food and produce vitamins - which are taken up by the body - as well as gases.

Step 5: Defecation

Body parts involved: Rectum

Any left-over material from the small intestine can now be considered as faeces (poo) once it reaches the large intestines which is approximately 6 feet in length. It comprises of six segments: the caecum, ascending colon, transverse colon, descending colon, sigmoid colon and the rectum. It is important to understand these segments as each one can be affected with disease and in some conditions like ulcerative colitis can determine the type of ulcerative colitis and what treatments options can be considered.

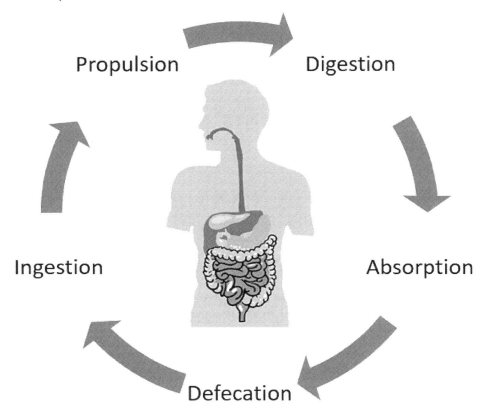

Once all the waste material has reached your rectum, which is the last part of your large intestine, are you able to defecate. Defecation occurs due to peristalsis, and similar to how the oesophagus moves food down towards the stomach, wave like contractions in the colon is able to push and move faecal matter towards the rectum. Your rectum has a number of receptors that can detect the presence of faecal matter and send signals to initiate a bowel motion.

How do we poo?

The act of expelling faecal matter from out digestive tract is called defecation and it is not as simple as just sitting down on the toilet and doing your business. Defecation is a complex process that involves not only the gastrointestinal system but the nervous and musculoskeletal system as well. This is because all these systems communicate with each other in order to tell each other what is going on in certain areas of the body. The process and maintenance of normal bowel movements requires the rectum to fill up with faecal matter and the body to be aware of this filling in order to set forth a number of signals that co-ordinate pelvic floor muscles, anal sphincter and rectal curvatures to expel faecal matter out.

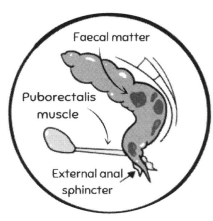

There are two main sphincters involved in the process of defecation: the internal and external anal sphincters. When the rectum fills up with faeces this causes it to distend which initiates the relaxation of a reflex known as the recto- anal inhibitory reflex (RAIR) which is mediated through the enteric nervous system. The RAIR is what keeps the anal sphincter closed when we do not need to defecate and so once this reflex is inhibited it causes the relaxation of the internal anal sphincter and gives the sensation of needing a poo. But it is not just the presences of poo in the rectum that is detected but also gasesas well, and there are secondary sensory mechanisms which are not yet well understood which help us determine if what is in our rectum is poo or just gas. If we are in a situation where going to the toilet is not convenient the feeling of needing to defecate initiates the voluntary contraction of the external anal sphincter until the feeling of needing a poo dissipates as the rectum relaxes. This allows more poo to be stored giving us a bit more time to find a toilet to relieve ourselves. Once we find a toilet and are sat on it a number of processes happen.

First, and most of the time we do not realise we do this, we hold our breath slightly which causes our diaphragm to contract activating our abdominal and rectal muscles which then causes the simultaneous relaxation of the external anal sphincter and the pelvic floor muscles. These process cause pressure to build to generate a pushing force that allows the anus to open to so defecation can occur.

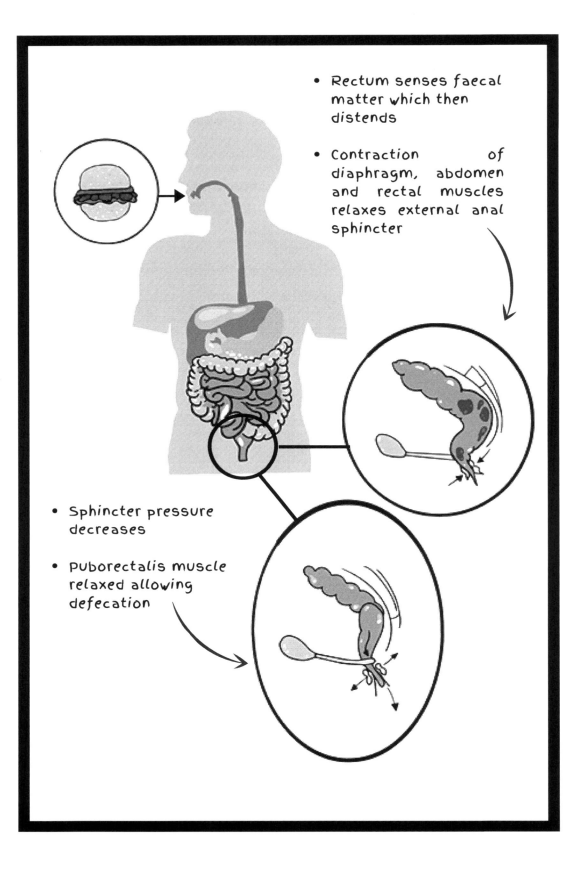

- Rectum senses faecal matter which then distends

- Contraction of diaphragm, abdomen and rectal muscles relaxes external anal sphincter

- Sphincter pressure decreases

- Puborectalis muscle relaxed allowing defecation

Often or not most of us are sit on the toilet hunched over scrolling through our phones and while for the majority of people this is allows for a normal bowel movement, for others this can actually prevent them from defecating. This is because their anorectal angle is not straight and one way to overcome this is change your position on the toilet which can be helped by using a defecation postural modification device (DPMD) which is essential a little stool (no not that kind of stool!).

A DPMD can help straighten out the anorectal angle as it mimics the normal position of squatting to defecate but on the toilet. You do not have to have a DPMD but can use a footstool instead while ensuring:

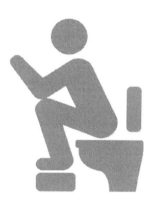

- Feet spread wide while on the footstool
- Ensure knees are slightly higher than your hips
- Lean slightly forward with elbows on your knees
- Keeping your back straight

However, our sitting position is not the only thing that can make defecation problematic. There are a number of issues which people with IBD experience due to their disease of which we will look at in more detail in chapter 6.

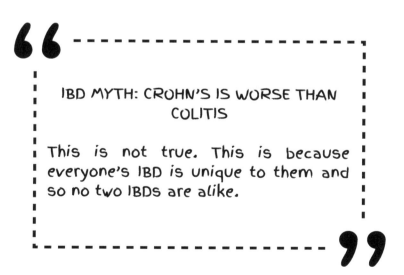

IBD MYTH: CROHN'S IS WORSE THAN COLITIS

This is not true. This is because everyone's IBD is unique to them and so no two IBDS are alike.

The Gut Microbiome

I'm sure many of you would have heard of the terms **gut microbiota** and **gut microbiome** and assume that they are referring to the same thing. Well even though they are related they are actually referring to different things. When we speak about our gut microbiota what we are referring to is the unique collection of the trillions of different microorganisms (bacteria, archaea, viruses and other microbes) in our gastrointestinal tract whereas the gut microbiome is referring to the entire environment (the gut) where these microorganisms are found.

The gut microbiota plays a vital role in human health as they assist in the following:

- **Nutrition:** The main food source for your gut microbiota is from dietary carbohydrates from indigestible **oligosaccharides** through the process of fermentation. This usually takes place in the large intestines and the gut microbiota are involved in carbohydrate, protein and fat metabolism where they are able to synthesis essential vitamins such a vitamin K and B vitamins which are important for our overall health. Additionally, and for example, a by-product of this fermentation process is a substance called oxalate, which if too much accumulates in the body can lead to kidney stones. There are certain bacteria within our gut that can counter this and help reduce the risk of kidney stones occurring which is an important consideration for some conditions as for example people with IBD are more at risk of developing kidney stones.

- **Drug Metabolism:** The medication we take can have an impact on our gut microbiota which are, believe it or not, also involved in how our bodies are able to process our medications and how effective those medications are. It is thought that the gut microbiota is able to convert **xenobiotic** drugs into their active forms and in doing so can impact on the **therapeutic efficacy** of that drug. As a result, many drugs that are for oral use are designed to not only withstand the transit through the gastrointestinal tract but are designed to make use of the gut microbiota to convert the drug from its inactive form to its active form. For example, Sulfasalazine is used in the treatment of IBD, and it has been designed to use specific enzymes found in certain bacteria found in the colon to produce sulfapyridine and 5-aminosalicylic acid, which have anti-inflammatory actions in the body, to help reduce the inflammation within the intestines due to IBD.

- **Immunity:** The gut microbiome has been associated with a number of chronic conditions such as IBD, colorectal cancer and irritable bowel syndrome (IBS), which has raised the question as to what the link is between the gut microbiota and human health. The gut microbiome is involved in both systemic innate and adaptive immune functions within the body and the aforementioned conditions are thought to cause an imbalance in the microbiome diversity that can lead to reduced immune tolerance. There are a number of bacteria within the gut that have been identified as key modulators of immune cells that help in maintaining the barrier function of the gut and protect against **pathogens** as well as being involved in inducing anti-inflammatory **cytokines** that help protect against diseases. For example, it is thought that a number of bacteria within the gut have anti-inflammatory properties and are able to protect against mucosal inflammation by producing anti-inflammatory cytokines and some studies have shown that some of these bacteria are in low in numbers in people with IBD.

There are however a number of additional factors that can have an impact on the gut microbiota:

- **Diet:** What is known as 'the western diet' is linked with many health conditions such as obesity and consists of primarily processed, readymade and fast foods all of which are high in salt, fat and low in dietary fibre. It is thought that this type of diet could be a contributing factor in the development of IBD, however there is insufficient evidence at this moment in time to make any definitive conclusions. Despite this, it is known that diet can alter the behaviour of our gut microbiota as they are able to adjust their metabolism depending on what type of food source is available to them, which can contribute to an imbalance in beneficial and 'bad' gut bacteria as well as causing changes to metabolic and inflammatory pathways within the body.

- **Disease:** Having an infection that affects the gastrointestinal tract is one of the most common causes of microbial imbalance in the gut. Pathogens that affect the gut can compete with the bacteria already present for space which can induce inflammatory responses which destabilises the gut microbiota causing symptoms such as bloating and diarrhoea. There is growing evidence to suggest that in someone with IBD, their genetics can make them more susceptible in developing IBD based on how their genes regulate the epithelial barrier of their gut and their immune response to microbial invasion of the gut. This in combination of the idea that external factors that cause alterations in the gut microbiome causing dysbiosis being involved in the pathogenesis of IBD.

- **Medications:** In understanding how drugs interact with the gut microbiota can help in furthering our understanding of how certain side effects from medications can be brought about. For example, antibiotics main purpose is to destroy a specific type of bacteria that causes you illness. However, the use of broad-spectrum antibiotics which are designedto target many different types ofbacteria increase the chances of disrupting the gut microbiota leading to dysbiosis. However, it's not just antibiotics that can have an impact on the gut microbiota but other medications as well and it is thought that some of the side effects, we experience from medication could actually be due to an imbalance in out gut ecosystem.

IBD MYTH: FATIGUE & TIREDNESS ARE THE SAME THING

This is not true. Fatigue can be difficult to describe and does not go away after a good night sleep or going to bed early.

- **Age:** After we are born the first thing that helps shape our gut microbiota is either breast milk or formula milk or a combination of both, depending on which one is used, will vary the number of bacteria that are dominant in the gut. This is important to understand as the development of the microbiota from a young age could play a vital role in not just the development of the infants' immunity but could impact on health later on in life. The process of getting older can also have an impact on our gut microbiota but the actual microorganisms in our gut do not age but they do get altered over time and it is still unclear if this alteration is due to or an implication of just getting older. However, ageing looks different for everyone as there are a number of other factors that can influence this process and the gut microbiota such as our diet and lifestyle choices.

"I was so shocked and so embarrassed at my symptoms that I didn't tell anyone hoping that everything would resolve on its own and eventually go away."

- **Stress/Anxiety:** To keep things simple there is something called the gut-brain axis which is a complex bi-directional communication between the gut and the brain involving the **hypothalamic pituitary adrenal axis** (HPA). Exposure to stressful events that may or may not cause a degree of anxiety can impact on the gut microbiota by altering the proportions found which can then influence the signals that are sent to the brain in response to these events. This can bring about symptoms experienced in IBD and IBS such as bloating, constipation and diarrhoea.

- **Exercise:** Participating in physical activity can positively influence the gut microbiota and can help in reducing the time taken for stool to move in your bowel and has additional benefits for your overall health and not just your gut health. In some studies, they found those that participated in exercise displayed increased levels of beneficial bacteria within the gut as well as the presence of **butyrate** (which has anti-inflammatory properties) that promoted overall good gut health.

> ## IBD MYTH: CROHN'S & COLITIS ARE THE SAME THING
>
> Even though they are types of IBD they are actually not the same. Crohn's disease can appear anywhere along the digestive tract whereas ulcerative colitis only affects the large intestine.

WHAT IS IBD?

There's a chance that some of you reading this may only have a rough idea of what IBD is.

There are two well-known forms of IBD, crohn's disease and ulcerative colitis, of which both are life-long conditions characterised by the inflammation of the gastrointestinal tract.

The exact cause of IBD is unknown but it is thought that a combination of a person's genetic make-up, atypical immune response and environmental triggers may play a role. Both are diagnosed and treated in similar ways and at the moment, there is no known cure for IBD, with current treatments being used to help reduce and manage symptoms.

The main feature of IBD is inflammation and ulceration of the digestive tract and depending on the location of this inflammation will determine the type of crohn's disease or ulcerative colitis an individual may have, the symptoms experienced and the severity of those symptoms will be dependent on how severe the inflammation and ulceration is.

There are however, in certain cases where clinicians cannot diagnose either crohn's disease or ulcerative colitis despite the symptoms being present in a person. In this case a diagnosis of indeterminate colitis is given which is sometimes known as IBD-unclassified, which despite being somewhat controversial is still a distinct clinical entity in itself.

Additionally, microscopic colitis can be considered as another form of IBD although it is not very well known and it is a condition where people often express chronic non-bloody diarrhoea as a symptom. There are two types of microscopic colitis (collagenous and lymphocytic colitis) and these conditions cause inflammation of the intestinal walls which can only be seen under a microscope, hence the name microscopic colitis.

TYPES OF CROHN'S DISEASE

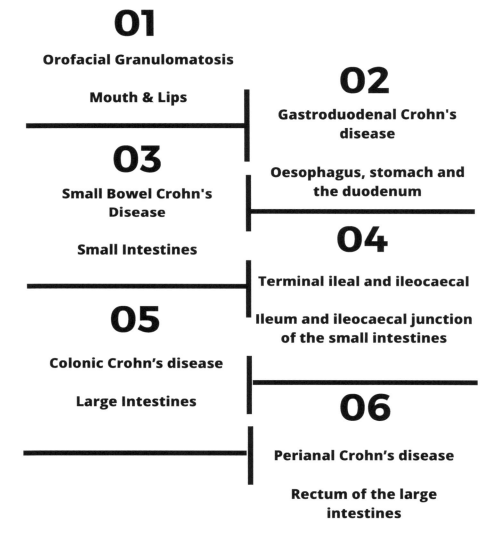

01

Orofacial Granulomatosis

Mouth & Lips

02

Gastroduodenal Crohn's disease

Oesophagus, stomach and the duodenum

03

Small Bowel Crohn's Disease

Small Intestines

04

Terminal ileal and ileocaecal

Ileum and ileocaecal junction of the small intestines

05

Colonic Crohn's disease

Large Intestines

06

Perianal Crohn's disease

Rectum of the large intestines

What are the symptoms of IBD?

Symptoms of crohn's disease and ulcerative colitis are the same however, even though people with IBD will experience the same types of symptoms the severity, frequency and order in which the symptoms will appear in will be different which adds to the challenge of diagnosing IBD.

The main symptoms of IBD include:

- **Pain:** This is such a non-specific symptom as anything can cause stomach pain and not just IBD. Experiencing frequent stomach pain which is alleviated after a bowel motion can be an indication of IBD.

- **Change in bowel habit:** This can vary from experiencing diarrhoea or constipation, but if you notice that your 'regular' bowel habit has changed and you are either going to the toilet more often or are struggling to have bowel motions then this could also be a sign.

- **Blood in stools:** Bleeding after a bowel motion should not be ignored as it could be a sign of IBD or something more serious and requires the immediate attention from medical professionals. Sometimes blood is not always present or noticeable if you have IBD as it depends where the bleeding occurs in your intestine. Bleeding that occurs higher up in the intestine can be the same colour or darker than stool as it has had time to congeal, whereas bleeding in the lower portion hasn't which is why it can be seen. You may find the blood is accompanied with either pus or mucus.

Types of Ulcerative Colitis:

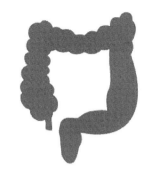

Total Colitis/Pancolitis

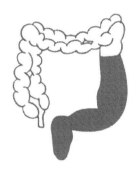

Left-sided Colitis

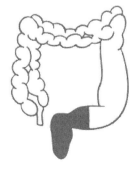

Proctitis

> **IBD MYTH: IT'S OK TO HAVE A LITTLE BLOOD IN YOUR STOOLS IF YOU HAVE IBD**
>
> This is not true. Even the presence of a little blood could be an indication that your IBD is active and so it is important to notify your doctor about this.

- **Loss of appetite and weight loss:** Some people can start to develop food avoidance behaviours as they associate food with pain causing them not to eat as well as losing interest or desire to eat food which can contribute to weight loss.

- **Iron deficiency anaemia:** Due to the nature of the IBD it can cause an impairment in how nutrients are absorbed by your body and so you may not be able to get all the nutrients you need which results in nutritional deficiencies. Iron deficiency anaemia can be caused due to nutritional deficiencies as well as excessive blood loss after each bowel motion.

- **Fatigue:** Every symptom of IBD mentioned previously can contribute to fatigue. Pain can interrupt sleep, using the toilet multiple times a day can be physically draining especially at night, nutritional deficiencies and blood loss can also deplete energy reserves.

> **IBD MYTH: PEOPLE WITH IBD ARE FUSSY EATERS**
>
> This is not true. While some people with IBD may avoid certain foods because they know it can trigger their symptoms, this does not make them fussy eaters.

How is IBD diagnosed

Most of the test and examinations conducted to obtain a diagnosis of IBD will also be done to help in the monitoring and surveillance of the condition. Some diagnostics tests provide more value and information than others but the most common ones conducted are:

Radiology:

- **X-Rays:** There are two types of plain film radiographs: abdominal x-rays or barium studies. Abdominal x-rays won't show IBD but they can show some of the complications of IBD such as bowel obstructions or perforations. Barium studies involved drinking a special drink that contains barium which then coats the digestive system as it travels through. This then allows either plain film x-rays or fluoroscopic real time pictures to be taken to show any abnormalities within the digestive tract.

- **Computed Tomography (CT) Scan:** CT scans can be described as a big round doughnut that often gets confused with magnetic resonance imaging (MRI) machines. CT scans are able to take 3D images of the internal organs and there are certain signs that can be looked for that can indicate intestinal inflammation as well as showing some of the complications of IBD such as fistulas, abscesses and strictures.

- **Magnetic Resonance Imaging (MRI) Scan:** MRI scans look similar to CT scans however they are very narrow and restrictive in space and so people can often find they get claustrophobic. MRI uses powerful magnets instead of radiation to get detailed images of the internal structures and can also pick up signs of intestinal inflammation and the complications of IBD.

- **Ultrasound Scan:** This type of scan uses sound waves to produce images and is often used in imaging pregnant women to monitor the health of their unborn child. It is quick, easy, painless and does not involve the use of radiation and can be helpful in showing some of the complications of IBD such as fistulas, intestinal narrowing and abscesses.

Endoscopy:

Endoscopy is the general term used to describe the use of a thin flexible tube with a camera attached to it to look at the internal health of the digestive tract. There are different types of endoscopic procedures all of which look at different parts of the digestive tract:

- **Colonoscopy:** This procedure will require the use of laxatives and to follow a special diet beforehand in order to empty your bowel. Duringthis procedure the endoscope will be passed through the anus to allow the entirety of the large intestine to be visualised in real time. During this procedure pictures, biopsies and samples from the colon are taken and the colonoscopy can be done under anaesthesia or lightsedation.

- **Flexible sigmoidoscopy:** This is similar to a colonoscopy apart from this procedure will only look at the last portions of the large intestine known as the rectum and sigmoid colon.

- **Gastroscopy:** In this procedure the endoscope will be passed through the mouth and down the oesophagus in order to look at the health of the stomach and first portion of the small intestine (the duodenum). This procedure can also be done under sedation for comfort purposes.

- **Capsule endoscopy:** This is a new type of technology where a pill that contains a camera is swallowed. The individual would be attached to some equipment which will help monitor the progress of the pill that was swallowed which will take pictures at intervals as it moves around the intestines allowing the doctors to then review the images.

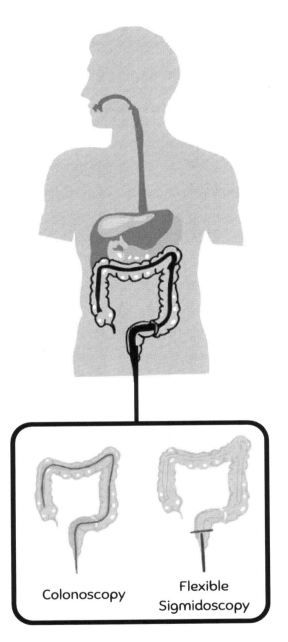

Colonoscopy   Flexible Sigmidoscopy

Blood Tests

Even though a blood test alone will not give a definitive diagnosis of IBD they can provide some indication that something may not be quite right by looking at certain levels within the blood by running the following tests:

- **Ferritin & Transferrin Test:** These tests look at the amount of ferritin (a protein that stores and releases iron) and transferrin (a protein that assists in in the transport of iron around the body) are in the blood.

- **Vitamin B9 & B12 test:** Vitamin B9 is also known as folic acid and vitamin B12 is also known as cobalamin. Folic acid works together with vitamin B12 in the formation of new red blood cells and vitamin B12 is needed for the normal function of our nervous system and formation of new red blood cells as well as for the metabolism of folate.

Low levels of folic acid and cobalamin due to blood loss and impaired nutrient absorption due to intestinal inflammation of IBD can cause both iron deficiency and vitamin B12 deficiency anaemia.

- **Inflammatory Markers:** An indication of inflammation within the body is high levels of C-reactive

protein (CRP) which is a protein made by the liver when inflammation occurs. Anything can cause CRP to be raised but very high levels, in combination with presenting with the other symptoms of IBD can be indicative of IBD.

Low levels of ferritin and transferrin can be an indication of iron deficiency anaemia which can be caused by blood loss and impaired nutrient absorption due to inflammation.

- **Full Blood Count:** This is a standardised blood test that can look at the overall health of an individual and looks at the amount of red blood cells, white blood cells and platelets within the blood. Low or high levels of these cells can be an indication of disease or deficiencies.

- **Erythrocyte Sedimentation Rate (ESR):** This tests the time taken for red blood cells (erythrocytes) to fall to the bottom of a test tube within an hour. Red blood cells should fall down slowly but when inflammation is present in the body other proteins can cause erythrocytes to fall down more quickly.

- **Liver Function Tests (LFTs):** This test measures how well the liver is functioning by looking at certain enzymes that are involved in many different processes in the body. People with IBD can have problems with their liver due to the medications that they are taking or abnormal LFTs can be an indication that inflammatory processes may be occurring within the body.

How is IBD Treated?

When it comes to prescribing medication or deciding which non-pharmacological approach to take for IBD, it is important to remember that these interventions will not cure IBD as there is no known cure as of yet.

As a result, the following interventions are designed to reduce the symptoms an individual is experiencing:

In people with IBD they are likely to also have Primary Sclerosing Cholangitis (PSC) which is a disease of the liver and gallbladder.

- **Aminosalicylates:** These are also known as 5-ASAs and are often the first type treatment people with IBD go on as they aim to help maintain remission and help prevent flare-ups. However, they are being used less and less for people who have crohn's disease as evidence suggests that they may not actually be of any help in the inducing remission. Some aminosalicylates like mesalazine come in different formulations and forms such as tablets, granules or enemas as each one is designed to be released and work on different parts of the digestive system. The type of 5-ASA an individual will go one will depend on the location and severity of the inflammation within the intestine.

- **Biologics:** Biological drugs used to treat IBD include infliximab, adalimumab, ustekinumab, vedolizumab and golimumab. They can get often get mixed up as they all sound similar but essentially the "mab" in the drugs name means they belong to a group of drugs that use mono-clonal antibodies. Mono-clonal antibodies are man-made antibodies that act like the ones found naturally in our immune system and these drugs are all designed to work on specific immune processes within the body that regulate inflammatory responses in order to reduce the inflammation of IBD.

IBD vs IBS

Many of you may have heard the terms IBD and IBS being interchanged for one another as if they were the same thing. While it is true that both present with similar symptoms, can be triggered by similar things, they are however not the same.

IBD is classified as an actual disease that causes intestinal destruction due to inflammation while IBS is defined as a syndrome or a disorder of gut function brought about by the control of the gut-brain axis (GBA). Furthermore, the differences don't stop there as you can actually see IBD when diagnostic imaging (x-ray, CT, MRI and ultrasound scans) are used whereas you can't see IBS on these scans and IBD is associated with an increased risk of developing colon cancer whereas IBS is not.

Even though symptoms of IBS (bloating, abdominal pain, diarrhoea and constipation) are like IBD, there are so many other features that separate the two. For example, IBD is associated with fatigue, weight loss, generally feeling unwell, loss of appetite as well as mouth ulcers whereas none of these are present in IBS. The most obvious difference between the two is that the extent of 'inflammation' in IBS does not compare to that seen in IBD in addition to there is no bleeding after bowel movements in IBS unlike in IBD further differentiating the two.

This then does bring into question as to how IBS symptoms are able to occur?

This isn't a simple answer as such as it is important to first to understand the Gut-Brain-Axis (GBA). The nervous system is made up of about one hundred billion cells called neurons which transfer signals received from within the body or the outside environment to the brain and back to the body. This allows the brain to control processes such as our breathing and helps us respond to things that can cause us pain. The nervous system is additionally split into two categories: the central nervous system (CNS) and the peripheral nervous system (PNS). The CNS is made up of the brain and spinal cord which are protected by the skull and the spine, whereas the PNS consists of all the other neurons in the body (not contained in the skull and spinal cord) and both the CNS and PNS have voluntary and involuntary mechanism known as the autonomic nervous system (ANS) and the somatic nervous system (SoNS). The ANS controls all the

- **Immunosuppressants:** These are drugs that suppress or weaken the immune system. As IBD is thought to be an autoimmune condition where the immune system of the host attacks itself causing inflammation, these drugs suppress the immune system in order to prevent it from doing any more damage to the body. Examples ofthese drugs include azathioprine, methotrexate and mercaptopurine and the doses that individuals will be on will depend on the severity of the intestinal inflammation.

- **Nutritional Therapy:** There are two types of nutritional therapy that can be used to help in treating IBD. Exclusive enteral nutrition is also known as the liquid diet and involves giving the bowel a break from food by using specially formulated drinks that provides the individual with all the nutritional sustenance they need instead of food. This is usually the first option for children who have IBD as the side effects are almost non-existent in comparison to corticosteroid treatment which can affect children's growth and development. The other type of nutritional therapy is called parenteral nutrition which involves the delivery of nutrition directly into the bloodstream via a cannula in the vein in the arm. This is often used after bowel surgery or if EEN is not working.

- **Corticosteroids:** These are often referred to as 'steroids' should not be confused with body building steroids and the ones used to treat IBD are known as corticosteroids. They work by reducing the activity of cells found in the immune system that activate inflammatory responses and examples of these drugs include budesonide, prednisolone and prednisone. These steroids are not used for the maintenance of long-term remission in IBD but rather deployed as a short-term strategy to help get individuals stable enough to be put on other medications.

- **Surgery:** There are many different types of surgical interventions that can be used to help in the treatment and management of IBD. Surgeries for IBD include surgeries to treat fistulas, abscesses, strictureplasty, bowel resections (ileocecal resection, limited right hemicolectomy and colectomy with ileo-rectal anastomosis), and stomas (ileostomy, colostomy, colectomy with ileostomy, proctocolectomy with ileostomy). Not everyone will require surgery and not everyone will have the same type or success rate from surgery as it will all depend which parts of the intestines are inflamed; how severe the inflammation is and the overall health of the individual.

> **IBD MYTH: EVERYONE WITH IBD WILL NEED TO HAVE A STOMA**
>
> Not true. Even though the majority of people with IBD will need to have surgery at some point, they will not all require a stoma.

> **IBD MYTH: IBD & IBS ARE THE SAME CONDITION**
>
> Not true. Even though they have similar symptoms, they are not the same and are claddified as seperate conditions

> **IBD MYTH: HAVING IBD MEANS YOU WILL GET CANCER**
>
> False. Having IBD can increase the risk of developing colorectal cancer, but this doesn't mean you will definitely get it.

the involuntary or subconscious process of the body such as our breathing, and to make things even more confusing, the ANS is further divided into the: the sympathetic (SNS), parasympathetic (PSNS) and enteric nervous systems (ENS).

For the purposes of IBS, the focus from this point onwards will be on the SNS, PSNS and ENS to understand how IBS symptoms are brought about. To keep things as simple as possible, the SNS and PSNS have opposing effects on the organs of the body. The SNS controls the parts of the body that prepares it for either physical or mental activity, such as increasing your heart rate or by decreasing the quantity of digestive juices released. The PSNS regulates the processes of the body that are used at rest and thereby decreasing the heart rate, relaxing muscles and increasing the quantity of digestive juices released. These processes are better known as part of the 'fight or flight' response.

The 'fight or flight' response is an acute physiological change that is brought about by a threat, that will allow the body to react to that threat by either staying to fight that threat or run away (flight) from it. These 'threats' cause the SNS to increase your heart rate, breathing rate and blood pressure to increase the supply of blood, oxygen and hormones to our brain and muscles to carry out a response. The SNS will also cause a decrease in the activities of non-essential systems or processes, such as digestion and the immune system, to deliver more energy to the components that are going to allow you to either fight the 'threat' or run away from it. When the threat is over, the PSNS can take over to return the body to its normal state by counteracting the effects of the SNS. In terms of IBS, these threats can include events that cause stress or anxiety which stimulate the 'fight or flight' response.

The third component of the ANS is the ENS which refers to the digestive tract that has neural components within it to allow the SNS and PSNS to trigger its activity. The gut is often described as the second brain and that is due to these neural components that it has so it has the capability to regulate the performance of the gastrointestinal tract without any help from the brain. Some studies have proposed that the brain is more of a receiver of signals rather than a transmitter when it comes to gut-brain communication. The gastrointestinal tract is made up of more than a thousand different microbes (**archaea, bacteria, eukaryotic** micro-organisms and **viruses**) that contribute to the metabolic and immune regulation of the gut by responding to physiological stimuli. The collection of these microbes within the human gut is given the name the gut-microbiome of which can communicate with the brain via the GBA. The GBA is the name given to interaction of the CNS, ANS, ENS and the hypothalamic pituitary adrenal axis (HPA). This communication is done through a complex network of special fibres of CNS structures and projections of the gastrointestinal tract muscle walls allowing the brain to regulate gut function and vice versa which is why it is known as a bi-directional communication network.

The HPA has three components: the hypothalamus, pituitary and adrenal glands. IBS is thought to be brought about due to exposure to external factors that induce stress and anxiety in an individual. Experiencing a stressful event or being put under pressure can activate the 'flight or fight' responses and causse the hypothalamus to release corticotropin-releasing factor (CRF), stimulating the anterior (front) portion of the pituitary gland to release adrenocorticotrophic hormone (ACTH). ACTH then causes the release of cortisol from the adrenal glands triggering the gut to release mast cells instigating the release of systemic proinflammatory cytokines. While this is occurring, both neural and hormonal forms of communication are occurring to allow the brain to influence the activity of the intestinal cells which also influences the gut-microbiome.

This process can indirectly cause the gut-microbiome to alter the activity and permeability of the gut, making it more or less active and allowing more of less water in thereby causing the common symptoms seen in IBS.

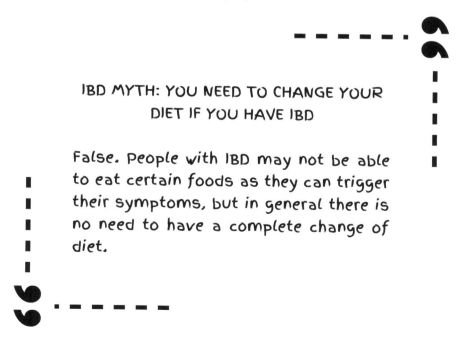

IBD MYTH: YOU NEED TO CHANGE YOUR DIET IF YOU HAVE IBD

False. People with IBD may not be able to eat certain foods as they can trigger their symptoms, but in general there is no need to have a complete change of diet.

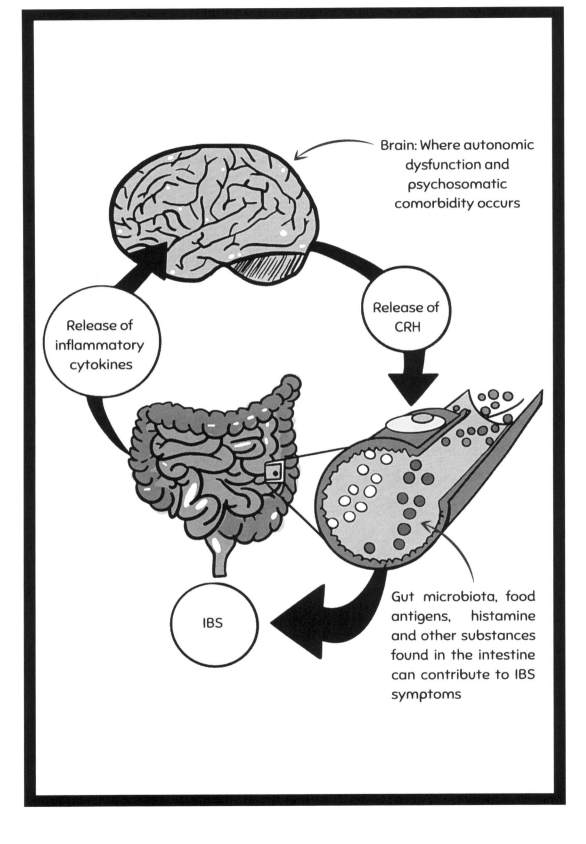

Brain: Where autonomic dysfunction and psychosomatic comorbidity occurs

Release of CRH

Release of inflammatory cytokines

Gut microbiota, food antigens, histamine and other substances found in the intestine can contribute to IBS symptoms

IBS

HOW IBD IMPACTS ON NUTRITION

When nutrition is spoken about, it is referring to the intake of food that is required to meet the energy demands of the human body. Eating well and having a well-balanced diet is important for good overall health and when combined with physical activity can help strengthen your immune system and improve physical and mental health.

However, with certain conditions like IBD, this can be a problematic because digestive tract disorders can lead to malnutrition. In the general population malnutrition is a term used to describe poor nutrition in an individual and it can refer to either not getting enough nutrients (undernutrition) or ingesting more than the body requires (overnutrition). Both can be very harmful to the body and there is no 'one size fits all' with nutrition as each person is unique and has different energy demands in addition to differences in the presence or absence of disease that impact on health.

When speaking about malnutrition in IBD, undernutrition is what is usually being referred to and it is seen more in crohn's disease than to ulcerative colitis, as crohn's disease can impair the ability of the small intestine leading to malabsorption of nutrients. The provision of nutritional care in IBD patients is of utmost importance to be able to prevent both macro and micronutrient deficiencies and despite each individuals' nutritional requirements being different the basic principles of what constitutes a healthy diet are the same:

- Eating at least 5 portions of fruits and vegetables a day
- Reducing the amount of saturated and trans-fats in our diets replacing them with polyunsaturated fats
- Reducing the amount of sugary and salty foods in our diets such as ready meals, sweets and fizzy drinks

What are nutrients?

The food we eat provide us with a variety of different nutrients (macronutrients and micronutrients) all of which play a role in the contributing energy to the body to allow it to carry out the essential functions such as growth, maintenance and repair.

Macronutrients are the nutrients that are needed in large amounts in our diet and consist of carbohydrates (sugars, starches and fibre), fats (monounsaturated, polyunsaturated, saturated and trans fats) and protein all of which are needed to provide a certain percentage of energy intake.

Micronutrients are the nutrients (vitamins and minerals) that are needed in small amounts and these are the substances that allow our body to carry out essential chemical reactions and other processes such as growth and development.

Some people with IBD may lack the enzyme called lactase which is needed to break down the sugar lactose.

This can cause them to be lactose intolerant which can cause bloating, stomach pains and diarrhoea.

The use of steroidal treatments in both adults and children with IBD can cause a loss in protein which is why some people are given elemental or polymeric supplements.

These liquid supplements contain easily digested nutrients, which also contain amino-acids or whole proteins, and come in different flavours.

Macronutrients

Carbohydrates:

These are the primary energy source for the body and not only do they help regulate blood glucose and insulin metabolism but provide at least over half the daily energy we require. They are also involved in cholesterol and triglyceride metabolism, and help with fermentation processes within the body.

Resistant starch is a type of starch that has the qualities of both soluble and insoluble fibre. It cannot be broken down by the small intestines as it acts like insoluble fibre here where it gets passed onto the large intestines. Once in the large intestine it acts like soluble fibre and is **fermented** by the bacteria within the colon who use it as a source of energy. Fibre is important for our digestive system as it acts as a

---

Why are carbohydrates important?

All the carbohydrates that you eat will get broken down by your body into glucose, which is a sugar that is easily used by our body to provide the energy we need to carry out our daily tasks.

Carbohydrates provide 3.75 calories per 1 gram and help to prevent the body using protein as a source of energy as protein is required for other vital functions such as growth and repair of the body.

Fibre contributes 2 calories per 1 gram and is a type of carbohydrate that is found in plants which the body finds difficult to digest and can be classified as either dietary fibre or resistant starch. Soluble fibre can help slow down digestion as it is able to dissolve in water and create a gel like substance. This allows it to be digested by the gut-microbiota providing them with a source of energy that allows them to increase in number. Insoluble fibre is not easily broken down by the gut-microbiota and acts as a bulking agent making our stools softer and easier to get rid of.

bulking agent preventing constipation. Fibre can also contribute to lowering the risk of developing heart disease, diabetes and colorectal cancer.

— 66 ——

People with IBD can find it difficult to incorporate certain foods into their diet for several reasons and so may not get enough carbohydrates causing the body to use fat stores as an energy source.

—————— 99 —

> ### *How they carbohydrates digested?*
>
> *Carbohydrates are first broken down by salivary amylase in our mouths. Here complex carbohydrates are broken down into smaller fragments and continue to do so for a time in the stomach, before the amylase is inactivated by the HCl present in the stomach. Any remaining carbohydrates must wait until they reach the duodenum of the small intestines where more amylase is secreted as a component of pancreatic juices, breaking them down into disaccharides. In combination with pancreatic juices, the presence of enzymes such as maltase, sucrase and lactase, in the small intestine can break down maltose, sucrose and lactose into glucose molecules respectively.*

Fats

Fat molecules are made up of fatty acids (a hydrocarbon chain attached to a carboxyl group) and glycerol (a small molecule with 3 hydroxyl groups) via a process called dehydration synthesis, where the hydroxyl groups on the glycerol react with the fatty acids. This will determine their chemical structure and depending on their chemical structure determines if they are either saturated or unsaturated fats. When we talk about the chemical structure of fats, what we are referring to is the length of the fat and its degree of saturation. A saturated fatty acid has all of its carbon atoms attached (or saturated) to hydrogen atoms and forms straight chains which means it has a high melting point. Unsaturated fatty acids are where the carbon atoms are not saturated with hydrogen because they have a double bond and can be monounsaturated (single carbon bond and the inclusion of a double bond between the two carbon atoms) or polyunsaturated fatty acids (PUFA) (two or more carbon double bonds that cause a kink in the structure).

However, not all fats are created equal and some may do the human body more harm than good. Trans fatty acids are also known as industrial trans fats as they are made by a chemical process that hardens vegetable oils. This process involves hydrogenating the vegetable oil and often described by using the term 'hydrogenated oil or fat' and can be found in takeaways, cakes, biscuits and fried foods. Trans fats do occur naturally in food, but only in very small amounts and low-level consumption of trans fats is unlikely to cause any long-term harm, however, the consumption of high levels of saturated and trans fats have been associated with high cholesterol and increasing the risk of heart disease. By reducing the amount of saturated fats consumed and replacing them with

"You never notice how good food looks when you're all of a sudden not allowed to have it and how much of our lives actually revolve around it."

unsaturated fats can help in reducing and maintaining blood cholesterol levels and cardiovascular health.

Polyunsaturated fats are considered to be essential fatty acids because the body cannot make enough of them examples being linoleic acid (a precursor of omega 6 fatty acid) and alpha-linolenic acid (ALA) (precursor of omega 3 fatty acid), and so it is essential to obtain these from the diet.

> **There is a strong consensus among experts that a diet abundant in fruit and vegetables, omega-3 fatty acids, and low in omega-6 fatty acids is allied with a reduced risk of developing crohn's disease or ulcerative colitis.**

> **Recommendation 1 of the ESPEN practical guideline (2020) on Clinical Nutrition in inflammatory bowel disease**

> ### Why are fats important?
>
> *Fats are another source of energy for the body, providing 9 calories per 1 gram of fat. The body is also unable to make certain essential fatty acids that it needs to allow the body the function normally and fat is also an essential component of the body's cellular membranes.*
>
> *Any excess fat obtained from the diet can be stored as adipose tissue as an energy reserve while providing insulation as subcutaneous fat preventing body heat loss. Fats provide transportation for vitamins A, D, E and K in the body as they are only able to be absorbed in the body when fat is present in the diet.*

There are two types of PUFA, omega 3 and omega 6 fatty acids, and they differ in chemical structure depending on the location of the last double bond on the end of their methyl molecule.

These types of PUFA are incredibly important in human health as they are both involved in growth and repair processesin the human body and can help in the maintenance of normal blood cholesterol levels and the normal function and development of the heart, brain and eyes. As they are both precursors, they can be used to make other omega 3 and 6 fatty acids such as eicosapentaenoic acid (omega 3) and docosahexaenoic acid (omega 3) and arachidonic acid (omega 6).

How are fats digested?

The trouble with fats is that they are not very easy to digest because they are not soluble in water and it is only when the food we've eaten gets turned into chyme by stomach and passes into the small intestines can fats be digested. Fat digestion requires the presence of bile in the small intestines which is produced by the liver. Bile is secreted into the small intestines via bile ducts where it mixes with the fats that a present in the chyme forming an emulsion of fat droplets. This helps digestion of fats as it creates a larger surface area of so pancreatic lipases (enzymes from the pancreas) can break down fats.

During this **emulsification**, the bonds between the glycerol and fatty acids of the fat molecules are being broken and being separated into smaller molecules. The fatty acids and glycerol mix with the bile and its contents forming something called **micelles** as the individual fatty acid and glycerol molecules are not soluble in water. The formation of micelles is important as they then transport the fatty acids, glycerol, vitamins and cholesterol to the cells that line the small intestines where they can then be absorbed into the bloodstream.

Proteins

What are proteins?

Proteins are made up of amino-acids and every single protein is unique in length, shape and size depending on the amount and type of amino-acids they contain. There are 20 different types of amino-acids which can be classified as either essential or

> In people with IBD there can be an imbalance in the amount of protein that is being used by the body and the protein that is being taken in. This can be due poor diet, side effects of treatments or insufficient absorption through the gut due to diseased segments.

non-essential amino-acids depending if they can be made by the body or not. The body is not able to makesome of these amino-acids (essential amino-acids) and so they must be provided by the food we eat, whereas non-essential amino acids can be made by the body.

Why are proteins important?

You may have heard protein being called 'the building blocks of life' – yes cast your mind back to GCSE biology lessons – and to be fair, they do live up to that description as they are involved in nearly every process that helps the body to function.

They are usually described in accordance to the function that they provide:

- ***Immunity:*** *Antibodies help protect the human body by binding onto pathogens such as viruses and bacteria that can make us sick. IBD is considered an autoimmune disease, which means these antibodies that are designed to protect us start attacking the body causing damage.*

- ***Enzymes:*** *These proteins are used to carry out the chemical reactions in the body. Each enzyme is different in shape and can only be activated when a specific substrate binds onto it. Think back to your biology lessons with the 'lock and key theory' and where enzymes are also known as catalysts as they can speed up the chemical reactions that occur in our body.*

- ***Growth & Repair:*** *Protein is found everywhere in the body from our bones, muscles, skin, hair and nails providing a type of scaffold to build our essential structures. As a result, protein is used to help repair these structures if they get damaged.*

- ***Hormones:*** *Our body requires ways to communicate with itself and one way it does that is by using hormones which are released by endocrine glands into the blood to help the co-ordination of biological processes.*

- ***Energy:*** *Protein is another source of energy for the body, providing 4 calories per 1 gram of protein.*

As proteins are large molecules, they first need to be broken down into smaller pieces to be digested and absorbed by the body. During the process of digestion, the enzyme pepsinogen is involved in the breakdown of proteins within the stomach. The HCl within the stomach not only kills off any harmful bacteria we may have ingested but it converts pepsinogen into its active form (pepsin) where it is then able to break down proteins.

Once enough time has passed and the mixture of your stomach contents forms chyme and passed into the duodenum of the small intestines, the enzymes trypsin and chymotrypsin which are in their inactive forms are released into the duodenum as part of pancreatic juices from the pancreas where they are activated. These enzymes continue to breakdown the proteins within the chyme into smaller pieces using an enzyme called peptidases which breaks the peptide bonds that hold the amino-acids together.

Micronutrients

Micronutrients are the nutrients (vitamins and minerals) that are needed in small amounts by the body and they are the substances that allow the body to carry out essential chemical reactions and other processes such as growth development and help strengthen the immune system.

There is a strong consensus among experts that it is a good practice point to recommend that people with active IBD require more protein (1.2-1.5 grams per kilogram of body weight in adults) than that of the general population and that when in remission protein requirements are similar to that of the general population (1 gram per kilogram of body weight).

Recommendations 5A & 5B of the ESPEN practical guideline (2020) on Clinical Nutrition in inflammatory bowel disease

There is a strong consensus among experts that people with IBD should be tested for micronutrient deficiencies regularly with any deficiencies being suitably dealt with by providing supplementation.

Recommendation 6 of the ESPEN practical guideline (2020) on Clinical Nutrition in inflammatory bowel disease

Vitamin A: Contributes to the normal function of the immune system, improves eyesight in low light as well as being necessary for the structure and function of the skin, lungs and digestive system. Vitamin A can be stored in the body and pregnant women should avoid having large amounts of vitamin A (whether through supplements or eating liver products and pate) as it can be harmful to the unborn child. A deficiency in vitamin A can cause night blindness and cause the conjunctiva and cornea of the eyes to become dry in a condition known as **xerophthalmia**.

As vitamin A is absorbed in the ileum of the small intestines some people with IBD may not be able to absorb as much as they would normally either because of inflammation of the ileum or removal of it due to surgery.

> **IBD MYTH: CROHN'S DISEASE IS MUCH WORSE THAN ULCERATIVE COLITIS**
>
> This statement is actually false. IBD will affect everyone differently and their experiences will be different, as will the severity of the intestinal inflammation present.

Vitamin B: These vitamins are absorbed in the jejunum and ileum of the small intestines. If someone with IBD has active inflammation in these parts of the small intestines or has had parts removed due to surgery, then this can affect how much of these vitamins they can absorb. Deficiency in B vitamins can cause fatigue and tiredness, both of which people with IBD suffer from because of their condition. As blood loss is also seen in IBD, this can also contribute to fatigue and tiredness which is why it is important that enough vitamins are obtained through the diet and if necessary, via supplementation to contribute to formation of new blood cells.

There is a total of eight B vitamins each of which contribute differently to the health of the human body.

B VITAMINS

THIAMINE

Helps to break down the food we eat and convert that food into energy by acting as a co-enzyme in metabolic processes which convert carbohydrates into energy. It also helps in the maintenance of our nervous system.

RIBOFLAVIN

This is also a co-enzyme that is involved in several metabolic processes that helps release energy from carbohydrates, proteins and fats, to help transport iron around the body while contributing to the normal functioning of the nervous system, skin and eyes.

NIACIN

There are two types of niacin (nicotinic acid and nicotinamide) and they are both important for the health and maintenance of the skin, nervous and digestive systems.

PANTOTHENIC ACID

The main function of pantothenic acid is that it is needed in the formation of co-enzyme A and acyl carrier proteins that are needed for the synthesis, transport and break down of fatty acids allowing the release of energy from the food we eat.

VITAMIN B6

This is also known as pyridoxine and is needed to help break down glycogen, form new red blood cells, modify steroidal hormones and transport of iron within the body.

BIOTIN

Biotin is important as it is a precursor for several enzymes that are needed to help break down glucose, fatty acids and amino acids.

VITAMIN B12

This is also known as cobalamin and it is needed for the normal function of our nervous system, formation of new red blood cells and maintaining normal homocysteine levels.

FOLATE

This is also known as folic acid or vitamin B9 and works together with vitamin B12 in the formation of new red blood cells. It is also important during pregnancy as it can reduce the risk of neural tube defects occurring.

> There is a strong consensus among experts that in people with crohn's disease who are nutritionally deprived over a period of time and who receive enteral or parenteral nutritional therapy are at risk of fluid and electrolyte shifts known as refeeding syndrome and require interventions that pay particular attention to phosphate and thiamine.
>
> Recommendation 21 of the ESPEN practical guideline (2020) on Clinical Nutrition in inflammatory bowel disease

> There is a strong consensus among experts that it is a good practice point to recommend that people that folate and iron levels of IBD patients who are pregnant should be monitored regularly due to the risk of deficiencies occurring. There is a strong consensus among experts that people with IBD who are being treated with sulphasalazine and methotrexate should be given folic acid supplementation.
>
> Recommendations 37 & 38A of the ESPEN practical guideline (2020) on Clinical Nutrition in inflammatory bowel disease

> There is a strong consensus among experts that if more than 20cm of the terminal ileum is removed due to crohn's disease that vitamin B12 injections as a form of supplementation is recommended.
>
> Recommendations 36 of the ESPEN practical guideline (2020) on Clinical Nutrition in inflammatory bowel disease

> *Vitamin C is important for people with IBD who have just had surgery or suffer from fistulas, as not only does it provide protection against possible infections, but it can help in the promotion of wound healing.*

Vitamin C: Vitamin C is also known as ascorbic acid, which supports the immune system by providing protection against free-radicals and as it cannot be stored in the body whatever is taken up is used. Vitamin C deficiency can cause a condition known as scurvy.

Vitamin D: Vitamin D is a hormone precursor that regulates calcium and phosphorus metabolism and there are two forms of vitamin D (vitamin D2 and D3) and it is important for good bone, teeth and muscle health while also contributing to muscle strength. We can obtain vitamin D2 from the foods we eat as part of our diet, but vitamin D3 is produced via sunlight by our skin. The skin has a component called 7-dehydrocholesterol which is converted into vitamin D3 by the ultraviolet rays from sunlight. The amount of vitamin D3 that is made depends on the amount of sunlight we are exposed to. Deficiency in vitamin D can cause the poor calcification of bones and in children vitamin D deficiency can cause rickets and osteomalcia in adults.

Vitamin E: Vitamin E is a fat-soluble vitamin that contributes to the maintenance of our eyes and skin as well as being an antioxidant that helps to protect the cells in our body from free radicals. Deficiency in vitamin E usually occurs in people that have fat malabsorption which can be seen in IBD. This malabsorption of fats

> There is a strong consensus among experts that both children and adults with active crohn's disease and ulcerative colitis who are receiving steroidal treatment should have their vitamin D levels checked and supplementation to be given if necessary.

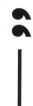

Recommendation 11 of the ESPEN practical guideline (2020) on Clinical Nutrition in inflammatory bowel disease

can cause fewer vitamins to be absorbed and can cause an increase in a substance called oxalate which can lead to kidney stones.

Vitamin K: Vitamin K is fat soluble which is needed by the body to help support the maintenance of healthy bones and blood clotting.

Minerals

Calcium: Calcium is an essential mineral as it contributes to the normal functioning of our vascular, nervous and skeletal systems. It contributes to building strong bones and teeth while helping our blood to clot normally after an injury. Calcium deficiency can lead to rickets in children as calcium is needed during ossification, and can lead to osteomalacia and osteoporosis in adults later in life.

Chloride: Chloride is involved in maintaining the balance of intercellular and extracellular fluid as well as in blood volume, blood pressure and pH in the body.

> There is a strong consensus among experts that both children and adults with active crohn's disease and ulcerative colitis who are receiving steroidal treatment should have their calcium levels checked and supplementation to be given if necessary.
>
> Recommendation 11 of the ESPEN practical guideline (2020) on Clinical Nutrition in inflammatory bowel disease

Fluoride: This is needed for the mineralisation of bones and teeth in the body and it is able to help protect against tooth decay.

Iron: Iron is important as it is a component of haemoglobin within the blood and it also plays an important role in many enzymatic reactions within the body including in the immune system as well as in the metabolism of energy and drugs within the body.

The lack of iron can impact greatly on your daily lifestyle causing low energy levels along with mental, sexual and physical impairment. Iron is one of many important minerals that we need to allow our body to function as it is one of the components of haemoglobin, that is found in red blood cells. One of the most common problems that is associated with IBD is anaemia, which is a term used to describe the decreased amount of red blood cells a person has. The name given to red blood cells is erythrocytes, and so the production of new erythrocytes is called erythropoiesis.

Haemoglobin is a metalloprotein (a protein that contains a metal ion (iron) cofactor), that gives blood its red colour which can transport oxygen to cells in the body and carry carbon dioxide to the lungs where it can be exhaled.

There are different types of anaemia, but iron deficiency is one of the most common problems associated with IBD. Men can be considered as being anaemic if they display haemoglobin levels of <140 g/L (<14 g/dL) where as a level of <120 g/L (<12 g/dL) is used for females.

The main reasons as to why iron deficiency is common in people with IBD is either due to or a combination of:

- *Inflammation of the intestines impairs its ability to be able to absorb iron (and other essential nutrients) causing there to be low levels.*

- *Not getting enough iron (and other nutrients) from the diet due to avoiding certain foods. This in combination with intestinal inflammation can contribute to iron (and other nutritional) deficiencies.*

- *The blood loss associated with IBD causes iron stores in the body to become depleted.*

The impaired absorption of iron and the loss of blood from gastrointestinal bleeding can limit the amount of iron that is available for erythropoiesis in those with IBD and this along with depleted iron stores in the body can easily lead to someone with IBD suffering from iron deficiency anaemia.

— 66 —

There is a strong consensus among experts that iron supplementation is needed in IBD patients who present with iron deficiency anaemia. Supplementation treatments will be determined on the level of deficiency with oral supplements being used first for those displaying mild anaemia with inactive disease. The use of intravenous iron can be the first line treatment offered in people who present with active IBD, previous intolerance to oral methods of supplementation or haemoglobin levels of <100g/L.

Recommendations 7A-C of the ESPEN practical guideline (2020) on Clinical Nutrition in inflammatory bowel disease

Magnesium: Magnesium contributes to the many functions in the body such as the activation of enzymes and hormones while being needed as a component which is involved in the cellular transport of calcium and potassium that contributes to the functioning of the nervous system by allowing our heart to beat and muscles to contract.

Phosphorus: Phosphorus works in combination with calcium in the formation of bone in the human body and there exists a dynamic equilibrium between calcium and phosphorus in adults when bone is remodelled. Phosphorus is also a component of the body's cells membranes as well as being involved in intercellular processes such as energy metabolism.

— 66 —————————

There is a strong consensus among experts that in people with crohn's disease who are nutritionally deprived over a period of time and who receive enteral or parenteral nutritional therapy are at risk of fluid and electrolyte shifts known as refeeding syndrome and require interventions that pay particular attention to phosphate and thiamine.

Recommendation 21 of the ESPEN practical guideline (2020) on Clinical Nutrition in inflammatory bowel disease

————————— 99 —

Potassium: Potassium is an electrolyte which contributes to allowing the electrical signals in the body to travel around and as it is not produced by the body so it is essential to obtain it from the diet to help in allowing the body to carry out its necessary functions. Deficiency in potassium can cause **hypokalaemia** which can lead to weakness, severe diarrhoea and even heart failure.

Selenium: Selenium is an antioxidant which can help protect against free radicals within the body that cause oxidative damage in addition to being involved in the immune system and reproductive function. Deficiency in selenium can cause Keshan disease which is a cardiac condition affecting mainly women of reproductive age and children whereas too much selenium can cause toxicity known as selenosis.

Sodium: Sodium is involved in the maintenance of normal cellular homeostasis and in controlling water and electrolyte equilibrium within the body and it is also important in the regulation of blood pressure, muscle and nerve conduction in the body and in the transport of nutrients in the body.

"Eating disorders are complex mental illnesses which can occur in anyone causing them to have an unhealthy attitude towards food"

*Sodium deficiency in the UK and other western countries is unlikely due to intake through diet being high. However, sodium deficiency (**hyponatremia**) can occur due to disease and other health conditions which then impacts the ability of the renal system to function.*

Zinc: Zinc is a cofactor in a number of enzymatic processes in the body and is involved in the metabolism of carbohydrates, proteins, fats while being an important component of cellular division, growth and repair. It also contributes in supporting the immune system, wound healing and reproductive function.

IBD MYTH: TAKING VITAMIN SUPPLEMENTS WILL CURE IBD

Unfortunately, this is not true. While taking vitamin supplementation can help in improving any deficiencies ibd you may have caused but it will not cure it.

There is a strong consensus among experts that in people with IBD who suffer with severe diarrhoea or who have high output with their ileostomy should have their fluid output and urine sodium monitored with the intention of adapting their fluid intake accordingly.

Recommendation 9A of the ESPEN practical guideline (2020) on Clinical Nutrition in inflammatory bowel disease

Pyridoxine is important for keeping blood homocysteine levels normal and people with IBD tend to have higher levels of homocysteine in their blood which is a risk factor for cardiovascular disease.

Probiotics & Prebiotics

Our gut is home to many kinds of bacteria that contribute to the health of our digestive system. The purpose of taking probiotics and prebiotics is to increase the number of these bacteria. A probiotic can be defined as a product that contains viable, defined microorganisms that are present in sufficient numbers that are able to alter the gut-microbiota and bring about beneficial effects within the host.

Prebiotics is another way of describing foods that have naturally occurring fibre such as fruits, vegetables, legumes, nuts and seeds.

These fibres cannot be broken down by our digestive system and so they are used as a food source by the bacteria found in our large intestines and as a result can influence the gut microbiota.

Are probiotics and prebiotics helpful in IBD?

The first thing to state is that there is no cure for IBD, however many people do find that taking both probiotics and

Probiotic Criteria

Not every microorganisms can be called a probiotic as they need to meet the following criteria:

- Be able to survive the stomach acid and reach the small and large intestines
- Must not cause harm to the host
- Be able to remain viable during the journey within the host
- Must be able to provide advantageous effects to host
- Has the ability to stabilise the gut-microbiome
- Can adhere to the intestinal lining
- Produce antimicrobial substances to harmful microorganisms

prebiotics helpful in either managing or alleviating their symptoms but it is important to discuss this and any form of nutritional supplementation with a registered dietician or nutritionist before starting on them. In the current scientific literature on it has been seen in children with ulcerative colitis that the use rectal enemas of *Lactobacillus reuteri* and the oral preparation of this probiotic (previously known as *VSL#3*) showed a moderate effect in two clinical trials. Recommendations of *VSL#3* only refer to the probiotic formulation which as from 2016 is no longer available under the brand name *VSL#3*. There are studies that have shown that *Escherichia coli Nissle 1917* strain and VSL#3 have benefited ulcerative colitis patients in

Naturally other probiotic formulations have been studied and despite being well tolerated by patient's significant effectiveness in inducing remission has not been shown while caution should be exercised in using *Lactobacillus rhamnosus GG* as there have been case reports of bacteraemia in patients with ulcerative colitis.

Other studies that have looked at the use of *VSL#3* in pouchitis noticed that using high doses of the probiotic *VSL#3* was effective in those that suffered with mild pouchitis whereas another study noticed promising results in achieving remission in mild to

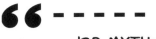

IBD MYTH: TAKING PROBIOTICS & PREBIOTICS WILL IMPROVE MY IBD SYMPTOMS

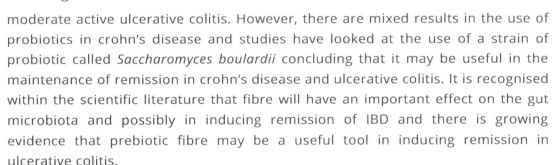

It is being recognised that probiotics can be helpful in those who suffer with IBS however there is limited evidence they are helpful in everyone that has IBD.

moderate active ulcerative colitis. However, there are mixed results in the use of probiotics in crohn's disease and studies have looked at the use of a strain of probiotic called *Saccharomyces boulardii* concluding that it may be useful in the maintenance of remission in crohn's disease and ulcerative colitis. It is recognised within the scientific literature that fibre will have an important effect on the gut microbiota and possibly in inducing remission of IBD and there is growing evidence that prebiotic fibre may be a useful tool in inducing remission in ulcerative colitis.

This was seen in some studies that showed promising results when fibre was added to the diets of ulcerative colitis patients, however given that the maintenance of remission was similar for germinated barley, *Plantago ovata seeds* and *Ispaghula husk* in these studies, it is thought that this is a generic effect of increased dietary fibre. In contrast, it is generally agreed dietary fibre may be unwise in IBD patients that suffer with intestinal strictures especially in those with crohn's disease. It is though that fibre in the form of prebiotic fructo-oligosaccharide is of no use in people with crohn's disease despite patients in some studies noting some benefit in taking wheat fibre supplementations and adopting an ovo-vegetarian based diet.

IBD MYTH: EVERYONE WITH IBD ARE UNABLE TO DIGEST SKINS OF FRUITS & VEGETABLES

Some people, such as those with an ileostomy, may find it hard to digest the skins of fruits and vegetables not everyone with IBD does. Some people with IBD may be advised to remove the skin from fruits and vegetables if they suffer with strictures or are currently in a flare-up.

Do Fermented Foods Help?

Fermented foods are foods or drinks that have been produced through the use of microbial growth and the anaerobic process of fermentation. During fermentation microorganisms like yeast and bacteria are able to break down components of food into other products, for example starch and sugar, and can be converted to alcohol or acids, while promoting the growth of probiotics.

While there is limited scientific evidence on the use of fermented foods in IBD, this doesn't detract from the fact that fermented foods can be used to provide a new dimension to the taste and texture of food. There are a number of additional health benefits that can be obtained from including fermented foods into your diet as these types of foods are often more nutritious in comparison to their unfermented states.

The process of fermenting food can make them easier to digest and the ingestion of probiotics formed during fermentation can help in reducing the effects of dysbiosis in the gut and help restore the balance of the gut microbiota alleviating symptoms often experienced by people who have IBS such as bloating, diarrhoea and constipation. Fermented foods are also rich in vitamin C, B vitamins and zinc which all contribute to the overall health of an individual as well as the functioning of the immune system.

"FOOD SHOULD TASTE GOOD AND IT'S MEANT TO NURTURE YOUR BODY & MAKING THIS SUBCONSCIOUS CONNECTION OF 'EATING MEANS BEING IN PAIN', I STARTED TO BECOME FUSSY ABOUT WHAT I ATE AND IN NO TIME AT ALL MY PERCEPTION OF FOOD CHANGED FROM FRIEND TO FOE".

Faecal Microbiota Transplant

Despite the exact cause of IBD being unknown the importance of the gut microbiota in IBD has been identified as vital. We know the gut microbiota is actively involved in the modulation of a number of physiological functions such as gastrointestinal and neurological development, immune response and resistance to pathogens. A healthy gut is characterised by the high levels of two major phyla, Firmicutes and Bacteroidetes which are underrepresented in people with IBD whose gut microbiome show high levels of facultative anaerobes from the phyla Actinobacteria and Proteobacteria.

Changes in the gut microbiota has been linked to intestinal inflammation due to dysbiosis of which is frequently observed in people with IBD causing a reduction in the microbes that produce anti-inflammatory compounds.

As a result, faecal microbiota transplant (FMT), which in simple terms is a poo transplant, has been looked at as a promising therapeutic option for those with IBD. Faeces from a 'healthy' subject is taken and all the beneficial bacteria and yeasts are extracted from it before they are transplanted into the colon of the recipient. While the earliest case report of FMT for IBD was reported in 1989 there have been studies that have showed its success in people who suffer from recurrent *Clostridium difficile* infection. However, despite data from clinical trials providing promising results it seems that FMT is more useful in those with ulcerative colitis than crohn's disease and that more research is needed to identify the most optimal route of administering FMT.

FMT can be administered either directly to the colon via colonoscopy, flexible sigmoidoscopy or an enema or it can be delivered through a capsule that is ingested. The risks of FMT in IBD aren't fully understood yet but risks that were seen for using FMT in those with recurrent *Clostridium difficile* infections included bowel perforation when colonoscopy was used as the delivery method.

Fluids

Alcohol

Alcohol is made up of carbon, hydrogen and oxygen atoms and is produced during the fermentation process between yeast and sugar. Alcohol is considered to be the second most energy dense 'nutrient' supplying 7 calories per gram but only a certain percentage of an alcoholic drink will be actual alcohol (strength) and so is known as alcohol by volume.

Adults over the age of 18 are permitted to drink alcohol, however UK government guidelines suggests that both men and women should consume no more than 14 units a week and that the consumption of alcoholic drinks do not count towards an fluid intake for the day. Alcoholic drinks can act as a diuretic and can increase fluid loss in urine and increasing the risk of dehydration. The negative consequences of excessive alcohol consumption on an individual's health is well documented but what is not well known is that chronic alcohol ingestion can impact on carbohydrate and fibre metabolism and inhibit the breakdown of triglycerides decreasing the quantity of free fatty acids in the body.

This can cause, even when macronutrient intake is adequate, blood glucose to rise or decrease and when there is no food to meet the energy demands of the body and stored sugar is depleted then by-products of alcohol metabolism can inhibit glucogenesis from other macronutrients like proteins. Despite alcohol being an energy source, its excessive consumption can also impair micronutrient intake indirectly as alcohol can inhibit fat absorption in which the knock-on effect is it impairs the uptake of fat-soluble vitamins.

It has been noticed in several studies that alcohol can worsen IBD symptoms and it is well known that the consumption of alcohol can alter the intestinal permeability.

It is thought that alcohol increases the risk of flare-ups by altering the luminal immune system, increasing the permeability of the intestines and increasing the exposure of the gut to antigens. The high sugar content of some alcoholic drinks is thought to cause osmotic diarrhoea which can contribute to gut dysbiosis.

While the impact of alcohol on IBD is being researched studies cannot identify a single specific alcoholic drink or the quantity that has the biggest influence on IBD symptoms.

Caffeine

Caffeine can be safely consumed but in moderation as excessive caffeine intake can have negative health effects causing an increase in anxiety, irritability, nausea, osteoporosis and sleep impairment. Caffeine also has diuretic effects and can increase a person's urine output increasing the amount of fluid lost by the body but this doesn't mean it will necessarily lead to dehydration.

In general it is important to remember to keep hydrated throughout the day and replace any fluids loss, however some caffeinated drinks like coffee can increase gastro-oesophageal reflux causing symptoms such as acid reflux, stimulate bowel activity and suppress appetite.

People with IBD can often suffer with acid reflux, over active bowels and have a loss of appetite and so while there is very little evidence in the literature to suggest that caffeine can cause or increase the risk of flare ups, current clinical guidelines suggest that people with IBD should try to avoid caffeine as a form of symptom management.

Water

The easiest way to obtain water and stay hydrated is to consume it in its liquid form, but we also obtain water from the foods we eat. It is recommended that on average we need to drink between 1.5-2Litres of water every day, however this figure will vary between individuals due to factors like activity levels and age. An estimation of fluid requirements of an individual can be made by following the formula of 1ml of water for every calorie an individual burn. For example, if a persons' calorie requirement for the day is 2,500 calories, then they should be aiming for 2.5 litres of water per day.

There are many different types of drinks in which we can consume however care should be taken as some drinks like fizzy drinks should be avoided or limited as they contain large amounts of sugar which can have negative consequences of general and oral health if consumed in large quantities regularly.

SIGNS OF DEHYDRATION:
- Extreme thirst
- Dry mouth
- Reduced urine output
- Feeling dizzy

DEHYDRATION REQUIRES IMMEDIATE AND URGENT MEDICAL ATTENTION FROM YOUR DOCTOR

Dietary Habits

In today's society, not only has gut health become an increasingly popular subject but so has the shift of focus on alternative and complimentary methods of treating disease. Food is no exception and there has been a recent change in belief that food can be used as a form of medicine and people with IBD have been seen to implement modifications to their normal dietary practices. IBD is known to cause loss of appetite and so this can impact on an individual's desire for food and so can have a knock-on effect on their social practices, like eating out with friends and family.

The one concerning fact about the access of readily available information from the internet is the risk of misinformation and lack of access to reputable sources, especially as many people are now self-prescribing dietary changes. There have been studies conducted that have shown people with IBD displayed changes in dietary behaviour pre and post diagnosis either as a way of providing symptom relief or to try and prolong their period of remission. Many people with IBD do recognise some foods as trigger foods as these foods either induce symptoms such as bloating, constipation or diarrhoea or can trigger a flare-up of their disease leading them to exclude these foods.

Often or not many people start to either exclude certain foods or entire food groups from their diet and while this is common practice amongst people who self-diagnose, it comes with many risks. We know IBD is associated with nutritional deficiencies which can impact on health and people who self-diagnose and self-prescribe dietary interventions are putting themselves at an increased risk of nutritional deficiencies.

Often or not many people start to either exclude certain foods or entire food groups from their diet and while this is common practice amongst people who self-diagnose, it comes with many risks. We know IBD is associated with nutritional deficiencies which can impact on health and people who self-diagnose and self-prescribe dietary interventions are putting themselves at an increased risk of nutritional deficiencies.

WHY THE INTEREST IN NUTRITION?

One of the reasons as to why I became so interested in the role of nutrition in IBD was because early on in my diagnosis I read several 'success stories' that claimed food can cure IBD and to someone in constant pain, anything that had the words 'cure for IBD' would inevitably catch my eye. The age-old questions you hear when it concerns IBD and food is either "can food causes IBD" or "can food cure IBD"? At the moment there is no evidence to suggest that food can either cause or cure IBD despite the number of cases of IBD in western countries increasing. This is leading some researchers to lean more on the theory that a western lifestyle – including diet – increases the risk of developing IBD.

"

IBD MYTH: DIET/FOOD CAN CAUSE & HELP CURE IBD

There is no cure for IBD however some people can find relief from avoiding certain foods that cause a trigger in their symptoms.

There is a strong consensus among experts that there is no specific diet that can help promote remission in either crohn's disease or ulcerative colitis patients with active disease.

Recommendation 8 of the ESPEN practical guideline (2020) on Clinical Nutrition in inflammatory bowel disease

"

IBD & The Western Diet

One of the main theories about what could possibly contribute to developing IBD due to gut dysbiosis is the adoption of the western lifestyle. This lifestyle includes changes in habits, urbanisation, industrialisation and dietary changes which are high in animal fat and low in fruits and vegetables and some studies have indicated that these factors are associated with an increased risk of developing IBD.

In comparison to other diets seen in the Mediterranean, Middle-East and Asia the components of the western diet contain a significantly higher proportion of calorie-dense industrialised foods which are high in saturated fats while being very low in fruits, vegetables and fibre. While the link between the western diet and obesity, cardiovascular disease and other non-infectious disease are well established, studies have also seen that the western diet increases intestinal inflammation due to dysbiosis. The link between the western diet and IBD is still being investigated but the association between the western diet and its components in eliciting either a direct or indirect intestinal inflammatory response is clear as day.

Furthermore, the western diet is very low in essential micronutrients that all contribute to everyday health and provide protection against disease by providing the body with substances that have both anti-inflammatory and antioxidant properties. Taking all of this into account it is not unreasonable to consider that a western diet could be a contributory component in the development of IBD.

However, it is unclear if there is a particular window of susceptibility to developing IBD in respect to exposure to the western diet whether during infancy, childhood or adulthood or if the chronic exposure to certain dietary components increase the overall risk.

Finally, when it comes to food, nutrition and even diets with IBD the fact remains that we are all different and have different preferences when it comes to food.

Trigger Foods

In today's society we are all obsessed about tracking how many steps we achieve in a day; how many calories are in the blueberry muffin we want but still avoid and we seem to analyses every aspect of our daily lives in the hopes to improve our health and well-being.

Taking note of our personal informatics can be useful and for those who have IBD and see a registered dietician are sometimes required to keep track of their dietary data in the hopes that it can shed some light on how to either prevent or manage their IBD symptoms.

Certain foods can cause people with IBD to experience a flare-up of their symptoms such as diarrhoea, constipation, bloating and nausea, with these foods being labelled as 'trigger foods' of which are usually foods that contain complex carbohydrates. The reason being is
that complex carbohydrates are harder to break down by the small intestines and so they are used as a food source by the gut microbiota in the large intestines causing fermentation.

This is a natural process that happens in everyone, however those with gastrointestinal disorders such as IBD can be very sensitive to changes in their gut-microbiota and consuming trigger foods can cause overgrowth of bacteria and yeasts that results in dysbiosis bringing about their symptoms.

There are a number of different types of hypersensitivities people can have with food and these include having food intolerances, allergies and psychological food aversions all of which differ from each other:

- **Food intolerances** involve a reaction being brought about by the body which does not involve the immune system when a certain food or component of food is ingested. For example, some people, including people with IBD, can be lactose intolerant meaning they do not have the enzyme called lactase. This enzyme is used to help break down the sugar lactose which is found in dairy products and those that are lactose intolerant are unable to break it down. This causes lactose to enter the large intestine where it is fermented by the bacteria in the colon causing bloating, wind, diarrhoea and abdominal pain.

- **Food allergies** are not the same as food intolerances. Having an allergy to food can be defined as an abnormal immune response to food or its components of which the level of the allergic reaction experienced can range from mild to severe which includes death. Some people can experience symptoms which involve the skin, gastrointestinal tract or the respiratory tract and any food can cause an allergy but the most common ones include eggs, peanuts, shellfish and nuts.

- **Food aversions** are a learned behaviour which can be brought about by a number of reasons such as associating specific foods (or food in general) with symptoms such as pain. Some can avoid foods based on the smell, texture and taste of the food or even can associate a type of food with a particular negative event or memory.

66 - - - - -

IBD MYTH: IBD IS CAUSED BY JUNK FOOD

There is little evidence to suggest that eating junk food is the sole cause of developing IBD. There is research being done on the link between IBD and the western diet.

- - - - - **99**

How to Identify Trigger Foods?

One of the easiest ways in identifying possible trigger foods is by keeping a food diary which can be analysed by a dietician or nutritionist and the way in which a food diary works is that it allows the tracking of certain aspects of your life which revolve around food.

Keeping an accurate food diary can help a dietician in identifying how balanced your diet is and seeing if you are getting enough of the essential nutrients your body needs to function. It also allows them to see what symptoms you were experiencing and after which foods and may encourage you to try excluding some foods or change certain eating habits to see if any benefit occurs from those changes.

WHAT TO WRITE IN A FOOD DIARY

 Time of day: Just writing down what you ate and how much you ate is not enough, as some people can find they get more symptoms eating at a certain time of the day.

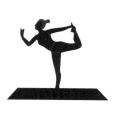 **Activity:** Eating while doing an activity such as watching TV, talking to friends or being alone can also play a part. For example, doing an activity such as watching TV or being in a rush to get somewhere can leave you distracted causing people to over eat, eat quickly, not chew food properly and ingest large amounts of air that can cause bloating later on.

 Mood: Your emotions also play a part in what you eat and how much of it you eat. Emotions such as stress, sickness, happiness can cause you to choose certain foods to either act as comfort or contribute to celebratory moods.

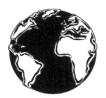 **Environment:** Environmental factors can influence what you choose to eat and drink and the quantity as well. It is important to note down where you were when eating these foods whether at home, at a friend's house or out at a restaurant.

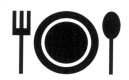 **Type of food/drink:** Write down what food and drink you had to during the day and how much of it you have had including any types of sauces or toppings.

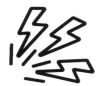 **Symptoms:** Writing down any symptoms you experience after sometime has passed since you've eaten and how bad they are can help in identifying trigger foods.

What IBD diets are there?

Despite there being an agreement by experts that there is no specific IBD diet that can be endorsed to help in establishing remission, this should not prelude the fact that when it comes to health and nutrition, we are all different. Just like treatments regimes for IBD being tailored to the need of the individual, nutritional approaches should also be the same with the help of a registered dietician or nutritionist.

The most common diets people with IBD follow are:
- **The LOFFLEX Diet:** The Low Fat, Fibre Limited Exclusion (LOFFLEX) diet was developed after it was noticed that patients with crohn's disease often exhibited a flare-up of symptoms once they ate foods that were high in fat and fibre. This dietary protocol involves the use of exclusive enteral nutrition to be used before hand in people with crohn's disease to try and achieve remission before following a food reintroduction plan eliminating food which are high in fibre and fat. It involves being supervised by experienced dieticians and nutritionists as a food diary is needed to be kept to note down any symptoms experienced while reintroducing food.

- **The Low FODMAP Diet:** People with IBD can also exhibit IBS-like symptoms even when their IBD is in remission and it has been suggested that diets which contain a high amount of fibre can bring about these IBS-like symptoms. The Low fermentable oligosaccharides disaccharides monosaccharides and polyols (FODMAPs) diet seems to be beneficial in people with IBS and as a result has gained a lot of attention with those that have IBD. FODMAPs are sugars that our gut finds difficult to break down with the majority being fermented in the large intestines. These sugars include fructose, lactose and polyols and they are a source of food for the bacteria in the large intestines with the by-products trigger symptoms like bloating, abdominal pain, diarrhoea and constipation. It should be noted that the relationship between FODMAP intake and inflammation of the intestine is unclear and that despite the possibility of gaining relief from IBS-like symptoms by following a low FODMAP diet, the risk of further nutritional deficiencies is high. This is because people with IBD are already considered as undernourished and nutritionally compromised due to their IBD and that the low FODMAP diet is very restrictive diet that can further compromise the health of the individual. If going on this diet, it is of vital importance that supervision and advice from a registered dietician or nutritionist is sought.

- **The Specific Carbohydrate Diet:** The concept behind the specific carbohydrate diet (SCD) is that it excludes more complex carbohydrates while only allowing the intake of simple ones as they are easier to digest. Complex carbohydrates tend to be poorly digested and so are used as a food source for the bacteria in the large intestine causing fermentation and overgrowth of bacteria and yeasts leading to dysbiosis and similar to the low FODMAP diet triggering symptoms. The SCD is not a form of low-carbohydrate diet, but instead it is a diet that is principally composed of monosaccharaides, solid proteins, fats, fruits, and nuts so that reduced amounts of disaccharide sugars are entering the large intestine. This is in the hope that any alteration in the gut-microbiota and dysbiosis is either prevented or reduced while still providing sufficient nutrition to the individual through the consumption of mainly monosaccharide sources such as fructose (found in fruits and honey), vegetables containing a higher amount of amylose, butter or oils, and solid proteins.

- **The Anti-inflammatory Diet:** The notion behind the anti-inflammatory diet (AID) is to reduce inflammation by consuming foods and spices that contain anti-inflammatory phytonutrients and omega-3 PUFAs. This is a diet that is rich in fruits and vegetables which are rich in antioxidants and even though animal proteins are allowed to be consumed this diet leans towards the consumption of plant proteins. There is a nutritional regimen of this diet in IBD patients and it is known as IBD-AID, which is derived from the SCD but it allows the consumption of grains and gluten making it less restrictive. IBD-AID also involves consuming omega-3 fatty acids and focusing on reducing the amount of saturated fats and has five basic phases to it.

The 5 Phases of the IBD-AID Diet

- **Phase I:** The modification of specific carbohydrates such as refined or processed complex carbohydrates
- **Phase II:** Emphasis on restoring gut-microbiota balance with the use of probiotics and prebiotics in the form of foods such as leeks, fermented foods and onions.
- **Phase III:** A focus on reducing the amount of saturated fats and eliminating hydrogenated oils while encouraging the uptake of foods rich in omega-3 PUFAs.
- **Phase IV:** To review the individuals overall dietary pattern and identify trigger foods, food intolerances as well as possible nutritional deficiencies.
- **Phase V:** The modification of food textures to encourage increased absorption of foods.

- **The Mediterranean diet:** This is closely related to the AID as it is focused on increasing the uptake of foods that are high in phytonutrients, unsaturated fats, omega-3 PUFAs, and wholegrains while decreasing the quantity of red meats consumed. It has been seen that this diet can contribute to the reduction of inflammatory markers within the body and appears as a promising medication free therapy for IBD. Foods consumed as part of the Mediterranean diet contribute to the health of the gut-microbiome and can reduce the risk of dysbiosis occurring while the intake of probiotic foods can help in restoration of gut-microbiota leading to improved gut health. Unlike the aforementioned diets the Mediterranean diet is less likely to contribute to the risk of nutritional deficiencies in people with IBD.

- **Gluten Free Diet:** People with celiac disease follow a gluten free diet (GFD). Celiac disease is an autoimmune condition where symptoms which include bloating, constipation, diarrhoea and nausea are brought about by eating foods that contain gluten. Gluten is an alcohol-soluble protein that is found in cereals, wheat, rye, barley and spelt and it is added to processed foods to help them maintain their shape.

The only treatment for celiac disease is to go on a GFD and some people with IBD can have an undiagnosed gluten sensitivity.

- **Palaeolithic Diet:** This diet is based on the idea that, as humans, we haven't changed much from our ancestors in the Palaeolithic era. This means this diet is based on the foods such as lean, non-domesticated meats and non-cereal plant-based foods of which our ancestors would have been able to obtain by hunting and gathering. It excludes processed foods, refined sugars, legumes, dairy, grains and cereals and promotes the consumption of grass-fed meats, fish, fruits and vegetables. The rationale here is that the prevalence of IBD is lower in rural areas where consumption of local produce is common practice.

IBD MYTH: I CAN'T EAT GLUTEN BECAUSE OF MY IBD

For some this can be true because some people with IBD can also have cealic disease and eating gluten can trigger symptoms. But for the majority with IBD there is no need to avoid gluten.

- **Plant Based Diets:** The attraction of plant-based diets (PBD) or the shift towards a PBD is gaining a lot of moment in modern society due to the perceived health benefits. These diets include going semi-vegetarian, vegetarian or even vegan and the idea behind them with IBD is to facilitate a move away from a westernised diet as studies have indicated diets high in animal fat and low in fruits and vegetables are associated with an increased risk of IBD. PBDs are thought to assist in gut microbiota **symbiosis**.

Stomas & Nutrition

A stoma is also known as an ostomy and it is the surgical method used to create an opening in the abdominal wall to allow a portion of the intestine to come through allowing it to excrete waste products. A bag (stoma bag) is fitted around this opening to collect the waste products and stomas are classified based on the segment of bowel that is brought to the outer surface of the body of which there are two types. An ileostomy involves bringing a segment of the small intestine through the abdominal wall whereas a colostomy involves bringing a portion of the large intestine through. There are a number of factors to considers when it comes to nutrition if you have a stoma as the

IBD MYTH: I NEED TO FOLLOW A SPECIFIC DIET IF I HAVE IBD

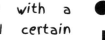

False. Everyone who has IBD will have different nutitional needs as the way their IBD impacts them and the medications their on is unique to them. Additionally, they will have their own personal religious and moral beliefs regarding food. This all will impact on the type and quality of food they are able to eat or diet they follow. Everyone is difference and so is the way we think, feel, behave around and digest food.

IBD MYTH: I NEED TO CHANGE MY DIET COMPLETELY BECAUSE OF MY STOMA

This is not true. While some people with a stoma avoid certain foods, which can cause blockages of the stoma or cause output (stool) to be watery or thick there is no reason to change your diet completely.

type of stoma that has been created will affect the body's ability to absorb nutrients, water and electrolytes and will also determine the consistency of the faecal matter excreted. With an ileostomy the whole on the large intestine is removed and a portion of the small intestine is brought to the surface, usually located on the person's right-hand side.

Having an ileostomy does decrease the ability of the body to absorb fluids, nutrients and electrolytes and the consistency of the stool produced will be determined on how much of the ileum is removed with thicker stool being an indication of absorbing more nutrients. Some people with an ileostomy can find it hard to digest foods rich in fibre and may find it best to avoid foods such as nuts and sweetcorn which can cause a blockage.

With a colostomy the small intestines are left untouched and depending on the severity and location of the inflammation in the large intestine will determine how much of it is removed.

People with a colostomy are still able to absorb most of their nutrients because the small intestines have been left untouched and depending on how much of the large intestines are removed might experience decreased fluid absorption.

In those with IBD and who have an *ileostomy* can find they are at more risk of dehydration because even though some water is absorbed through the small intestine the majority is absorbed by the large intestine. They may also find that they are unable to absorb sufficient levels of vitamin B12 which is primarily absorbed in the last portion of the small intestine and they may require vitamin B12 supplementation.

STOMA LIFESTYLE TIPS:

- Always speak to your dietician and stoma nurse about any concerns you have

- Ensure your stoma bag fits well to avoid the risk of contents leaking onto skin

- Emptying your bag regularly can help in avoiding leaks

- Don't skip meals as this can cause nutritional deficiencies and cause more gas to occur in the stomach.

- Try wearing loose clothing for comfort and to hide the outline of your bag

- Try and avoid odorous foods

- Ask your stoma nurse about sprays and powders that can neutralise odours

- Avoid fizzy drinks which can cause gas contributing to noises made by the stoma

- Reduce/Quit smoking as this can increase the amount of gas entering your bag

- Try and stay well hydrated throughout the day and avoid gulping your drinks

Nutritional Therapy

Exclusive Enteral Nutrition

This is also known as the liquid diet and is well established as a first line therapy for children and teenagers with crohn's disease. It is used mainly for crohn's disease because inflammation from the disease can affect the small intestines which is where the body absorbs all the essential nutrients from the food we eat and the inflammation can impair that ability. The use of corticosteroids is often preferred over EEN for crohn's disease, however there is a growing consensus that corticosteroids should be avoided in the first instance when it comes to the paediatric population.

IBD MYTH: I WILL BE ON THE SAME FORMULA FOR THE REST OF MY LIFE

This is not true. If you are having EEN the length of time you will be on it will vary and the type of drink you will be given will be based on your current health status. EEN formulas come in lots of different flavours to help in providing you with a variety of choice.

This is because the side effects of corticosteroids can impact on a child's growth, development and bone mineral density in addition to causing changes in body shape leading to incidental consequences, especially among adolescents, such as self-confidence and body image issues.

EEN involves the use of specially formulated liquid drinks that are designed to be exclusively used as a substitute to solid foods for between six to eight weeks. This form of therapy is designed to give the bowel a 'break' from the constant motion of mechanical and chemical digestion of food and to encourage the healing of the gut mucosa. It can be given orally or via a nasogastric tube. These specially formulated drinks consist of either polymeric, elemental or semi-elemental drinks all of which contain differing complexities of the essential macronutrients which we need. The type of formula that people with IBD will be given will be determined on an individual basis. EEN is a vital therapeutic option in the management of crohn's disease and while it is likely that it influences the gut microbiota reducing the dysbiosis seen in people with IBD its main advantage if it induces remission in children is that it avoids the unwanted side effects of medications such as corticosteroids. While it is uncommon for adults to be on EEN, it is used as a form of additional supplementation to diet.

Parenteral Nutrition

Parenteral nutrition which is what people with IBD will go on when they are unable to obtain enough nutrients from food and when EEN isn't an option or isn't working. It is the delivery of electrolytes, macronutrients and micronutrients through intravenous methods, bypassing the normal process of how food is absorbed from the gut and ensuring they go directly into the bloodstream. Just like EEN the reasons for and the duration of going on parenteral nutrition will be determined on an individual basis, but parenteral nutrition will be given to prevent malnutrition as the body can't get enough nutrients due to either the inflammation in the intestines or because of other complications of IBD. Parenteral nutrition can be delivered either by having a cannula inserted into a vein or have a peripherally inserted central catheter (PICC) line inserted. Having a cannula inserted is the simplest and this will be placed in the arm which will then be attached to a line that is connected to a special bag containing the parenteral nutrition formula. Having a PICC line inserted is a little a bit more complicated as it does require a minor procedure to be carried out. In general, either local anaesthetic or sedation will be given and a radiologist will insert a catheter into a vein in located on the arm and under x-ray guidance guide it into a large vein that carries blood to your heart. This line can also be used to administer medication but in this case, it will be used to deliver the parenteral nutrition. There are risks associated with having parenteral nutrition as the cannula insertion site of the PICC line itself could become infected as well as an allergic reaction occurring in people who have an egg allergy. This is because in some parenteral nutrition formulations there may be traces of egg. Additionally, because the nutrients are being directly administered into the bloodstream, salt and electrolyte levels will be closely monitored to make sure kidney and liver function is normal.

— 66 —

IBD MYTH: YOU CAN BECOME DIABETIC IF YOU GO ON PARENTERAL NUTRITION

One of the risks of parenteral nutrition is that it can make your blood sugar levels high as the formula contains a lot of glucose, it does not mean you will become diabetic. You will have your sugar levels monitored just in case you need insulin to manage it and that your levels should return to normal once parenteral nutrition has been stopped.

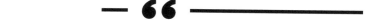

PARENTERAL VS ENTERAL NUTRITION

PARENTERAL NUTRITION

Parenteral nutrition designed to deliver nutrients to the body directly into the blood stream, thereby bypassing the conventional way of eating and digestion by the gut. It can be delivered by:

ENTERAL NUTRITION

Enteral nutrition is a liquid-based diet using specially formulated nutritional drinks that can be delivered orally by drinking or it can be delivered by inserting a:

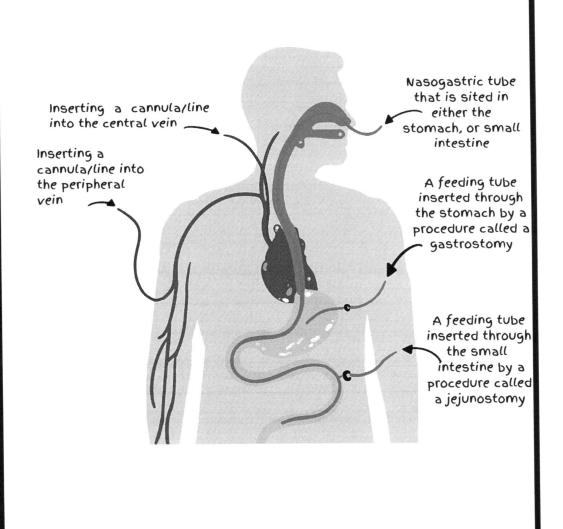

Inserting a cannula/line into the central vein

Inserting a cannula/line into the peripheral vein

Nasogastric tube that is sited in either the stomach, or small intestine

A feeding tube inserted through the stomach by a procedure called a gastrostomy

A feeding tube inserted through the small intestine by a procedure called a jejunostomy

INTESTINAL COMPLICATIONS IN IBD

Those with IBD can suffer from an array of complications which is determined by the location and severity of the inflammation in their gut of which can affect the way the gut works and can contribute to the symptoms experienced. The most common complications are:

- **Abscesses:** People with IBD are likely to develop abdominal or pelvic abscess throughout their life. An abscess is formed when the inflammation of IBD penetrates down deep into the wall of the intestine causing the area to become infected which results in the formation of pus. These can cause pain and fever and usually require a small procedure called a **percutaneous abscess drainage** to help drain the pus and treat the infected area. A further complication of having an abscess is that it can later on develop into a fistula.

- **Fistulas:** These are abnormal passages that occur either between two holloworgan and the body surface with the majority of fistulas in IBD occurring in the perianal region (anus) connecting to the surface of the anus. Depending onthe location of the fistula and what it connects to will determine the type of fistula present of which there are five types: **perianal** (anal fistula), **enterovesical** (bowel to bladder fistula), **enterocutaneous** (bowel to skin fistula), **enteroenteric** (bowel to bowel fistula) and **rectovaginal** (bowel to vagina) fistulas. There are many different ways in which fistulas can be treated such as using antibiotic, immunosuppressive and biologic medication however in most cases people will require surgical intervention such as having a fistulotomy, fistula plug, endorectal advancement flap, a ligation of intersphinteric fistula or having a **seton** inserted to drain away the pus that has collected.

- **Perforations:** A perforation is the term used to describe when a structure has ruptured or ripped. Bowel perforations in IBD are rare but can occur due to severe inflammation of the intestinal wall that causes a stricture which leads to an obstruction (blockage) instigating the bowel to perforate which require surgery to treat. Another complication relating to bowel perforations in IBD is toxic megacolon which is a rare life-threatening condition where inflammation causes the large intestines to swell and expand. It is described as a non-obstructive dilation of the large intestine and is usually associated with ulcerative colitis where gases produced in colon as part of normal digestion becomes trapped contributing to this swelling. This increases the risk of the large intestine perforating which is why development of toxic megacolon symptoms should not be ignored and urgent medical assistance should be sought out. Perforations in IBD (and in general) are dangerous as all the contents of the bowel will start to leak into the abdominal cavity leading to **sepsis** which is life-threatening.

SYMPTOMS OF TOXIC MEGA-COLON:

High temperature
Increased heart rate
Abdominal pain
Abdominal swelling

TOXIC MEGACOLON IS A SERIOUS MEDICAL CONDITION AND REQUIRES THE IMMEDIATE ATTENTION MEDICAL ATTENTION FROM DOCTORS

- **Strictures:** Inflammation of the intestines because of IBD can cause it to become damaged and so the body will naturally try to heal that damage. As the inflammation in IBD is chronic, this means the process of damage and healing is on a continuous cycle which leads to **fibrosis** of the intestinal walls. The formation of scar tissue at the site of damage in the intestine causes the affected area to start to become thick decreasing the size of the intestinal lumen which makes the diameter of the intestinal lumen to become much narrower than before. This is the stricture and it can make it difficult for digested food to pass through and start to cause symptoms such as abdominal pain and constipation. In some cases, this narrowing can be very severe that it can cause bowel obstructions which can lead to bowel perforations that would require emergency surgery to correct.

Constipation

Constipation can be defined as the inability to be able to pass stool or empty the bowel on a regular basis and is often accompanied by the need to strain when having a bowel motion due to stool becoming hard and dry. There are many causes of constipation which can include:

- Anatomical causes such as intestinal strictures, anal stenosis or atresia

- Side effect of drugs or even the use of recreational drugs can cause constipation

- Endocrine and metabolic disorders such as diabetes and hypothyroidism

- Abnormality in intestinal nerve functioning such as spinal cord defects or Hirschsprung disease

- Faecal withholding behaviours which can lead to a build-up of hard stool

In people with IBD constipation can be caused by inflammation of the rectum (proctitis), a low-fibre diet, dehydration, side-effects of IBD medications as well as damage to the anal muscles due to surgery.

CONSTIPATION TIPS:

- Speak to your doctor before taking any medications

- Increase fibre intake (this may not be advisable if you suffer with strictures)

- Laxatives can help in providing constipation relief

- Bulking agents can help soften hard stools

- Change your seating position on the toilet

- Stay hydrated by drinking plenty of water

- Try exercising as this can help increase gut motility

66

"I STILL REMEMBER THE CONSULTATION I HAD AND BEING TOLD THAT THERE WAS NO CURE FOR CROHN'S DISEASE AND IT REALLY FELT LIKE THE PROVERBIAL RUG HAD BEEN PULLED OUT FROM UNDERNEATH ME."

BLOATING TIPS:

- Speak to your doctor before taking any medications

- Consult a dietician to identify any food sensitivities/intolerances

- Look at eating habits and eating environment

- Avoid fizzy/carbonated, caffeinated and alcoholic drinks

- Reduce levels of stress

- Exercise frequently

- Wear loose clothing to alleviate pressure on your abdomen if you suffer from bloating

- Try drinking peppermint tea

- Drink plenty of water and stay hydrated

Bloating & Flatulence

Bloating is one of the most common issues experienced in people with IBD and IBS and can be defined as a sensation of gassiness or a sense of **distention** sometimes accompanied with visible increase in abdominal girth.

The severity of bloating and discomfort felt is determined by the amount of gas that has amassed in the intestines with a number of theorised mechanisms proposed as to that what causes gas production including:

- Carbohydrate fermentation by the gut microbiota
- Small intestine bacterial overgrowth (SIBO) a condition where excess bacteria within the small intestines produces gas
- Altered gut motility causing an impairment in the way gas is managed naturally within the intestines
- Irregularities in the abdominal-diaphragmatic reflex that impacts on normal gut motility
- Hypersensitivity of the abdominal viscera where the presence of normal quantities of gas are interpreted as bloating

- Carbohydrate malabsorption due to food intolerances such as lactose intolerance
- Distention of the rectum by retained hard stool causing constipation can slow down gut motility and cause the sensation of bloating.

Diarrhoea

Diarrhoea can be defined as having three or more loose or watery bowel motions in a day, and can be classified as either acute, chronic, infectious or non-infectious and occurs as a result of the impairment in the ability of the large intestine to absorb water. Acute diarrhoea can last less than two weeks and is usually caused by a viral or bacterial infection whereas chronic diarrhoea can last more than four weeks and is classified as non-infections as common causes include chronic disease like IBD or even side effects of medications.

Food intolerances and sensitivities can also be a cause of diarrhoea as some people are unable to tolerate certain foods. Some find that eating foods that are spicy, high in fat and that have lots of fibres can cause people with IBD to experience diarrhoea as it is thought that people with an irritable bowel have a higher number of nerve fibres in their bowel that react with spices compared to the general population. Additionally, fat malabsorption in IBD can contribute to diarrhoea as insufficient amounts of bile salts are absorbed back into the small intestines leading to a higher amount of bile salts entering the colon causing an increase in colon secretions, resulting in watery diarrhoea.

Extensive diarrhoea causing more fluid to be lost than what is being taken in can cause dehydration. This causes an imbalance of the electrolytes in the body with the most obvious sign of dehydration is feeling very thirsty, which is one way your body is telling you that it needs fluids.

Symptoms of dehydration can range from having headaches, a dry mouth, lack of energy and passing dark yellow urine. However, severe dehydration can present as spells of dizziness, pale and dry skin and getting muscle cramps, which requires immediate medical attention. Alcoholic beverages and drinks that have caffeine can contribute to dehydration as well. Staying well hydrated is not only important for the normal function of the body, but it also helps keep our stools soft making it easier to defecate. Becoming dehydrated can cause constipation as stool will start to dry up and become hard making it difficult to defecate.

DIARRHOEA TIPS:

- Speak to your doctor before taking any medications
- Anti-diarrheal drugs can be used to provide some relief
- Bulking agents can help in making stools thicker as well as softening hard stools
- Avoid certain foods that you know that can cause you to have diarrhoea
- Antispasmodic drugs can help in reducing the motility of the gut allowing more water to be absorbed
- Pack an emergency travel kit with baby wipes, spare change of clothes and toiletries
- Obtain a RADAR key which gives access to disabled toilets
- Wear incontinence products such as pads or underwear
- Try doing pelvic floor exercises to strengthen pelvic muscles

"Anyone with IBD who has lost weight can tell you it is the hardest thing to try and put back on no matter how much you eat and for years my weight and the topic of food has been such an issue."

In people with IBD who have frequent bowel motions can often find the presence of blood, pus or mucus in their stool and often experience diarrhoea during a flare-up. This is because the lining of the intestines becomes inflamed which compromises its functioning, alters the body's immune response and increases the number of antigens present in the intestines. The inflammation then this causes less water to be absorbed making stools waterier and loose resulting in a quicker transit time through the colon.

Faecal Incontinence

Faecal incontinence (FI) is defined as involuntary loss of either liquid or solid stool and is often an overlooked 'symptom' in people with IBD and is commonly known as frequent bowel movements, urgency or **tenesmus**.

The most commonly associated concern of FI is not being able to find or have readily available access to a toilet when out in public and so FI can have such a negative impact on a person's life. This fear of not being able to find a toilet when not at home can lead to social isolation, can impact employment status, sexual practices, as well as self-esteem and quality of life as people choose to avoid activities and leaving the house due to the fear of embarrassment if FI occurs.

FI is common in people with IBD who suffer with perianal fistulas or have an ileo-anal pouch but can also occur due to old age, in women who had complications during vaginal childbirth as well as to those who have had surgical procedures around the anus causing loss of the recto-anal inhibitory reflex.

FI can be treated surgically and non-surgically with the main goals being to improve a person's quality of life, improve stool consistency, reduce the amount of stool in the rectum and slow down bowel motility.

FI surgical intervention aims

- Correction of underlying abnormalities such as recto-vaginal and perirectal fistulas

- Using techniques like sacral nerve stimulation to improve functioning of the anal sphincter

- Repair the anal sphincter if it is damaged

- Replace or support the anal sphincter by using an artificial bowel sphincter or implantation of a pelvic sling system

- Divert the bowel by creating a colostomy

- Try to reduce faecal load using Malone antegrade continence enemas

FI non-surgical options:

- Antidiarrheal drugs

- Making dietary changes to avoid foods that trigger diarrhoea or increase bowel activity

- Increasing fibre intake or use of bulking agents (these may cause people with IBD to experience bloating and abdominal distention and so caution should be exercised)

- Physical therapy and biofeedback training can help strengthen pelvic floor and sphincter muscles.

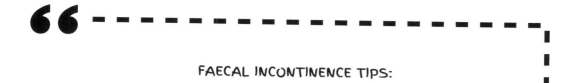

FAECAL INCONTINENCE TIPS:

- Speak to your doctor before taking any medications
- Pack an emergency travel kit with baby wipes, spare change of clothes and toiletries
- Obtain a RADAR key which gives access to disabled toilets
- Wear incontinence products such as pads or underwear
- Try doing pelvic floor exercises to strengthen pelvic muscles
- Avoid certain foods that you know that can cause you to have diarrhoea

Gastro-Oesophageal Reflux

Gastro-oesophageal reflux disease (GERD) is a common upper oesophageal condition that is characterised by heart burn and acid reflux as symptoms. The causes of GERD are multifactorial and involve different mechanisms:

- **Impairment of the lower oesophageal sphincter** (LES) is thought to contribute to GERD. The LES is located at the end of the oesophagus and acts as a gate way into the stomach. Above the stomach contents is a zone of high intragastric pressure with spontaneous moments of relaxation by the LES which facilitates in the venting of gases in the stomach. People who suffer with GERD have more frequent LES relaxation events which causes the intragastric pressure to increase to the point where the LES cannot contain it causing reflux of the stomach contents into the lower portion of the oesophagus.

- **Hiatal hernias** are commonly seen in people with GERD and the presence of a hiatal hernia impairs the ability of the LES to function properly and hindering its ability to keep the contents of the stomach in the stomach.

- **Impairment of oesophageal peristalsis** is also thought to be another cause of GERD. When we chew food our it is mixed with salivary bicarbonate in the mouth and when we swallow our food is able to travel down to our stomach due to wave like movements (peristalsis) pushing the food down the oesophagus. The normal functioning of our oesophagus along with salivary bicarbonate is able to clear and neutralise any reflux present, however in those with GERD this doesn't happen as often and so causes a build-up of gastric reflux due to decreased clearance.

Treatment for GERD

Treatment usually involves lifestyle and, in some cases, dietary changes with advice mainly focused on the reduction of cigarette and alcohol intake, avoidance of certain trigger foods in addition to weight loss and adaptation of sleep position.

GERD TIPS:

- Speak to your doctor before taking any medication

- Eat small and frequent meals

- Try keeping your head and chest above the *level of your waist* when lying down to prevent stomach acid travelling up your oesophagus

 - Avoid eating up to 4 hours before bed and avoid known trigger foods

- Try to quit or reduce intake of cigarettes and alcohol

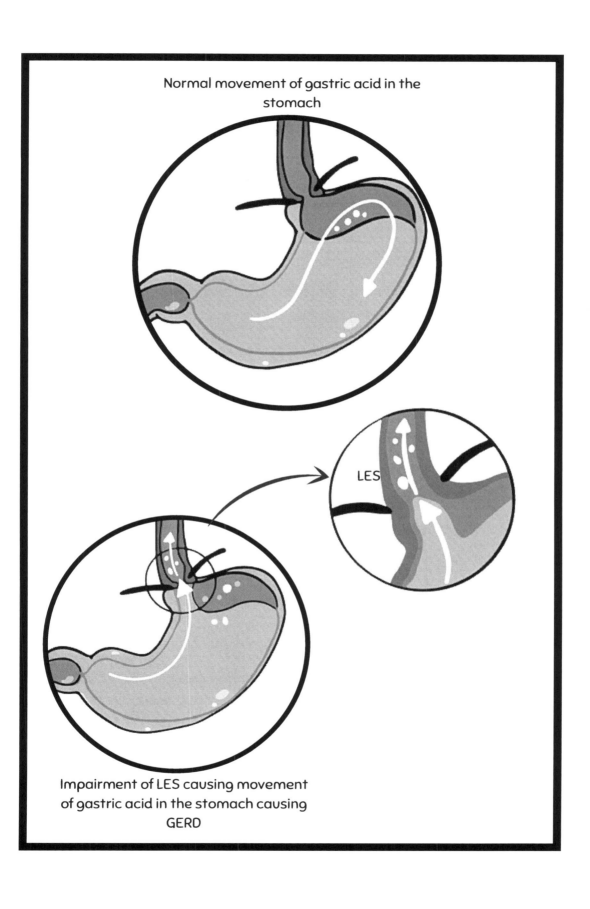

Normal movement of gastric acid in the stomach

LES

Impairment of LES causing movement of gastric acid in the stomach causing GERD

GLOSSARY

- **Atresia:** Atresia is a condition where an opening or passage way in the body is closed or absent.

- **Antibodies:** A protein found in the blood that is able to react to a specific antigen as part of the body's immune system.

- **Antioxidant:** A substance that is able to prevent oxidation in the body which can cause damage.

- **Archaea:** A microorganism that is similar to the size and shape of bacteria but is molecularly different.

- Avoidant/Restrictive Food Intake Disorder: A type of eating disorder where the individual avoids or restricts intake of certain foods or food in general.

- **Bacteraemia:** The presence of bacteria in the blood which can cause infection.

- **Bacteria:** A unicellular organisms that does not have cell walls and can cause some diseases.

- **Butyrate:** An ester of butyric acid that has anti-inflammatory properties.

- **Catalyst:** A substance that is able to speed up the rate of a chemical reaction but is not used up or changed during the process.

- **Chyme:** The name given to partially digested food before it enters the small intestine from the stomach.

- **Cortisol:** A steroid hormone made by the body which is involved in a number of different physiological process.

- **Cytokines:** A substance that is secreted by the cells of the immune system that can have an effect on other cells within the body.

- **Dehydration Synthesis:** A chemical reaction that involves joining two substances together by removing water.

- **Distention:** This is the enlargement or swelling of something. For example, abdominal distention refers to swelling of the abdomen.

- **Dysbiosis:** The imbalance in organisms found in an individual's microflora that can contribute to causing health conditions.

- **Electrolytes:** The ionised constituents of the blood (for example Na+ (sodium) and K+ (potassium).

- **Emulsification:** The mixing of two liquids which are not usually mixable to form an emulsion.

- **Endocrine glands:** A gland that is able to secrete a substance such as a hormone into the bloodstream.

- **Enterocutaneous Fistula:** An abnormal channel or connection that forms between the bowel or stomach and the skin.

- **Enteroenteric Fistula:** An abnormal channel or connection that forms between the bowel.

- **Enterovesical Fistula:** An abnormal channel or connection that forms between two sections of the bowel.

- **Eukaryotic:** An organism that has a nucleus in their cells enclosed by a nuclear envelope.

- **Fermented:** The name given when a substance has undergone the process of fermentation.

- **Fibrosis:** The medical term given to describe the thickening and scarring of tissue within the body.

- **Gut Microbiome:** The entire collection of microorganisms that are present in a person's gastrointestinal tract.

- **Gut Microbiota:** The individual microorganisms that are found in a person's digestive tract.

- **Gut-Brain Axis:** The name given to describe the bi-directional communication between the central nervous system (brain) and the enteric nervous system (gut).

- **Hirschsprung Disease:** A birth defect where a portion of nerve cells in the bowel are absent causing an impairment in gut motility.

- **Hypoglycaemia:** When blood glucose levels drops to low levels and mainly affects people with diabetes and can be dangerous if not raised to normal levels.

- **Hypokalaemia:** The name given when potassium levels are lower than 3.5mmol/L.

- **Hyponatremia:** The name given when sodium concentration in the blood is lower than 135mmol/L.

- **Hypothalamic Pituitary Adrenal Axis:** Also known as the adrenal axis which is the interaction between the hypothalamus, pituitary and adrenal glands to regulate the body's physiological responses to certain stimuli.

- **Hypothyroidism:** The medical term given to an underactive thyroid where it doesn't produce enough of the necessary hormones your body needs.

- **Keshan Disease:** This is a reversible disease of the heart muscles that is characterised by necrosis of heart cells and is associated with inflammatory infiltrates and calcification.

- **Mastication:** The name given to the process of chewing food.

- **Micelles:** These are fat molecules that form a spherical shape when in water.

- **Oligosaccharides:** Types of carbohydrates that are formed when three to ten simple sugar molecules are linked together in a chain.

- **Pathogenesis:** The term given to the development of a disease or condition.

- **Pathogens:** A substance such as a virus or bacteria that causes disease.

- **Percutaneous Abscess Drainage:** The use of diagnostic imaging to locate an abscess and insert instruments to drain the fluid out.

- **Perianal Fistula:** An abnormal channel or connection that forms between the anal canal and the perianal skin.

- **Peristalsis:** A series of wave like contractions that help food travel down the oesophagus as well as through the digestive tract.

- **Rectovaginal Fistula:** An abnormal channel or connection that forms between the rectum and the vagina.

- **Refeeding Syndrome:** The shift of fluids and electrolytes that can occur in malnourished patients receiving either enteral or parenteral nutrition which can be fatal.

- **Segmentation:** The combination of circular and longitudinal muscle movements in the digestive system and peristalsis in the small intestine to mix food and ensure it comes into contact with the intestinal walls to better assist in absorption of nutrients.

- **Selenosis:** Toxicity caused by the intake of too much selenium.

- **Sepsis:** This is a life-threatening condition whereby your body's immune system overreacts to an infection and causes damage to your internal organs.

- **Seton:** A piece of surgical thread or 'string' that is inserted into a fistula to help it drain allowing it to heal.

- **Stenosis:** This is the narrowing of a space. For example, stenosis of the intestines is referring to the narrowing of the intestine.

- **Symbiosis:** The interaction between two organisms that provides each other with a certain benefit.

- **Tenesmus:** This is the feeling of the need to defecate.

- **Therapeutic efficacy:** The medical term given to how well a medication or medical device designed to treat conditions help to improve that condition or disease.

- **Viruses:** A microorganism that causes disease by replicating itself once it has infected the hosts cells.

- **Viscera:** This refers to the main organs within the body.

- **Xenobiotic:** Refers to a synthetic or man-made chemical such as a drug that is foreign to the body of the individual that takes it.

- **Xerophthalmia:** The dryness of the conjunctiva and cornea of the eye caused by vitamin A deficiency.

REFERENCES

Chapter 1: Introduction

- Beat Eating Disorders (2020), Types of Eating Disorders, [Online] Available at: https://www.beateatingdisorders.org.uk/support-services/helplines

Chapter 2: Understanding the Gut

- Patricia JJ, Dhamoon AS. Physiology, Digestion. [Updated 2020 Aug 16]. In: StatPearls [Internet]. Treasure Island (FL): StatPearls Publishing; 2020 Jan-. Available from: https://www.ncbi.nlm.nih.gov/books NBK544242/
- Ogobuiro I, Gonzales J, Tuma F. Physiology, Gastrointestinal. [Updated 2020 Apr 16]. In: StatPearls [Internet]. Treasure Island (FL): StatPearls Publishing; 2020 Jan-. Available from: https://www.ncbi.nlm.nih.gov/books/NBK537103/
- Biga, L. M., Dawson, S. et al., The Digestive System Anatomy & Physiology. Pressbooks. Retrieved from http://library.open.oregonstate.edu/aandp/chapter/23-2-digestive-system-processes-and-regulation/
- Thursby, E., & Juge, N. (2017). Introduction to the human gut microbiota. The Biochemical journal, 474(11), 1823–1836. https://doi.org/10.1042/BCJ20160510
- Hills RD Jr, Pontefract BA, Mishcon HR, Black CA, Sutton SC, Theberge CR. Gut Microbiome: Profound Implications for Diet and Disease. Nutrients. 2019;11(7):1613. Published 2019 Jul 16. doi:10.3390/nu11071613
- Jandhyala, S. M., Talukdar, R., Subramanyam, C., Vuyyuru, H., Sasikala, M., & Nageshwar Reddy, D. (2015). Role of the normal gut microbiota. World journal of gastroenterology, 21(29), 8787–8803. https://doi.org/10.3748/wjg.v21.i29.8787
- Enright, E. F., Gahan, C. G., Joyce, S. A., & Griffin, B. T. (2016). The Impact of the Gut Microbiota on Drug Metabolism and Clinical Outcome. The Yale journal of biology and medicine, 89(3), 375–382.
- Durack, J., & Lynch, S. V. (2019). The gut microbiome: Relationships with disease and opportunities for therapy. The Journal of experimental medicine, 216(1), 20–40. https://doi.org/10.1084/jem.20180448
- Zuo, T., & Ng, S. C. (2018). The Gut Microbiota in the Pathogenesis and Therapeutics of Inflammatory Bowel Disease. Frontiers in microbiology, 9, 2247. https://doi.org/10.3389/fmicb.2018.02247
- Hasan, N., & Yang, H. (2019). Factors affecting the composition of the gut microbiota, and its modulation. PeerJ, 7, e7502. https://doi.org/10.7717/peerj.7502
- Zinöcker, M. K., & Lindseth, I. A. (2018). The Western Diet-Microbiome-Host Interaction and Its Role in Metabolic Disease. Nutrients, 10(3), 365. https://doi.org/10.3390/nu10030365

- Albenberg, L. G., Lewis, J. D., & Wu, G. D. (2012). Food and the gut microbiota in inflammatory bowel diseases: a critical connection. Current opinion in gastroenterology, 28(4), 314–320. https://doi.org/10.1097 MOG.0b013e328354586f

- Langdon, A., Crook, N., & Dantas, G. (2016). The effects of antibiotics on the microbiome throughout development and alternative approaches for therapeutic modulation. Genome medicine, 8(1), 39. https://doi.org/10.1186/s13073-016-0294-z

- Vich Vila, A., Collij, V. et al., (2020). Impact of commonly used drugs on the composition and metabolic function of the gut microbiota. Nature communications, 11(1), 362. https://doi.org/10.1038/s41467-019-14177-z

- Nagpal, R., Mainali, R., Ahmadi, S., et al, (2018). Gut microbiome and aging: Physiological and mechanistic insights. Nutrition and healthy aging, 4(4), 267–285. https://doi.org/10.3233/NHA-170030

- Appleton J. (2018). The Gut-Brain Axis: Influence of Microbiota on Mood and Mental Health. Integrative medicine (Encinitas, Calif.), 17(4), 28–32.

- Foster, J. A., Rinaman, L., & Cryan, J. F. (2017). Stress & the gut-brain axis: Regulation by the microbiome. Neurobiology of stress, 7, 124–136. https://doi.org/10.1016/j.ynstr.2017.03.001

- Monda, V., Villano, I., Messina, A., et al (2017). Exercise Modifies the Gut Microbiota with Positive Health Effects. Oxidative medicine and cellular longevity, 2017, 3831972. https://doi.org/10.1155/2017/3831972

Chapter 3: Overview of IBD

- Chang, C. W., Wong, J. M., Tung, C. C., Shih, I. L., Wang, H. Y., & Wei, S. C. (2015). Intestinal stricture in Crohn's disease. Intestinal research, 13(1), 19–26. https://doi.org/10.5217/ir.2015.13.1.19

- Richards R. J. (2011). Management of abdominal

- and pelvic abscess in Crohn's disease. World journal of gastrointestinal endoscopy, 3(11), 209–212. https://doi.org/10.4253/wjge.v3.i11.209

- Scharl, M., & Rogler, G. (2014). Pathophysiology of fistula formation in Crohn's disease. World journal of gastrointestinal pathophysiology, 5(3), 205–212. https://doi.org/10.4291/wjgp.v5.i3.205

- Lewis, R. T., & Bleier, J. I. (2013). Surgical treatment of anorectal crohn disease. Clinics in colon and rectal surgery, 26(2), 90–99. https://doi.org/10.1055/s-0033-1348047

- Fontana, T., Falco, N., Torchia, M., et al (2017). Bowel perforation in Crohn's Disease: correlation between CDAI and Clavien-Dindo scores. Il Giornale di chirurgia, 38(6), 303–312. https://doi.org/10.11138/gchir/2017.38.6.303

- Desai, J., Elnaggar, M., Hanfy, A. A., & Doshi, R. (2020). Toxic Megacolon: Background, Pathophysiology, Management Challenges and Solutions. Clinical and experimental gastroenterology, 13, 203–210. https://doi.org/10.2147/CEG.S200760

- Nemati, S., & Teimourian, S. (2017). An Overview of Inflammatory Bowel Disease: General Consideration and Genetic Screening Approach in Diagnosis of Early Onset Subsets. Middle East journal of digestive diseases, 9(2), 69–80. https://doi.org/10.15171/mejdd.2017.54
- Ranasinghe IR, Hsu R. Crohn Disease. [Updated 2020 Jun 9]. In: StatPearls [Internet]. Treasure Island (FL): StatPearls Publishing; 2020 Jan-. Available from: https://www.ncbi.nlm.nih.gov/books/NBK436021/
- Baumgart D. C. (2009). The diagnosis and treatment of Crohn's disease and ulcerative colitis. Deutsches Arzteblatt international, 106(8), 123–133. https://doi.org/10.3238/arztebl.2009.0123
- Tremaine W. J. (2011). Diagnosis and treatment of indeterminate colitis. Gastroenterology & hepatology, 7(12), 826–828.
- Storr MA. Microscopic colitis: epidemiology, pathophysiology, diagnosis and current management – an update 2013. ISRN Gastroenterol. 2013; Article ID 352718, 12 pages, 2013. doi:10.1155/2013/352718.
- O'Toole A, Coss A, Holleran G, et al. Microscopic colitis: Clinical characteristics, treatment and outcomes in an Irish population. Int J Colorectal Dis. 2014;29:799-803.
- Shor, Julia et al. "Management of microscopic colitis: challenges and solutions." Clinical and experimental gastroenterology vol. 12 111-120. 27 Feb. 2019, doi:10.2147/CEG.S165047
- Lamb CA, Kennedy NA, Raine T, et al British Society of Gastroenterology consensus guidelines on the management of inflammatory bowel disease in adults Gut 2019;68:s1-s106.
- Abdul Rani, R., Raja Ali, R. A., & Lee, Y. Y. (2016). Irritable bowel syndrome and inflammatory bowel disease overlap syndrome: pieces of the puzzle are falling into place. Intestinal research, 14(4), 297–304. https://doi.org/10.5217/ir.2016.14.4.297
- Akbar, A., Yiangou, Y., Facer, P., Walters, J. R. F., Anand, P., & Ghosh, S. (2008). Increased capsaicin receptor TRPV1-expressing sensory fibres in irritable bowel syndrome and their correlation with abdominal pain. Gut, 57, 923–929. https://doi.org/10.1136/gut.2007.138982
- Canero, E. M., & Hermitte, G. (2014). New evidence on an old question: Is the "fight or flight" stage present in the cardiac and respiratory regulation of decapod crustaceans? Journal of Physiology Paris, 108(2–3), 174–186. https://doi.org/10.1016/j.jphysparis.2014.07.001
- Carabotti, M., Scirocco, A., Maselli, M. A., & Severi, C. (2015). The gut-brain axis: Interactions between enteric microbiota, central and enteric nervous systems. Annals of Gastroenterology, 28(2), 203–209. https://doi.org/10.1038/ajgsup.2012.3
- Kennedy, P. J., Cryan, J. F., Dinan, T. G., & Clarke, G. (2014). Irritable bowel syndrome: A microbiome-gut-brain axis disorder? World Journal of Gastroenterology, 20(39), 14105–14125. https://doi.org/10.3748/wjg.v20.i39.14105

- König, J., Wells, J., et al.,(2016). Human intestinal barrier function in health and disease. Clinical and Translational Gastroenterology, 7(10). https://doi.org/10.1038/ctg.2016.54
- MacDermott, R. P. (2007). Treatment of irritable bowel syndrome in outpatients with inflammatory bowel disease using a food and beverage intolerance, food and beverage avoidance diet. Inflammatory Bowel Diseases, 13(1), 91–96. https://doi.org/10.1002/ibd.20048
- Major, G., & Spiller, R. (2014). Irritable bowel syndrome, inflammatory bowel disease and the microbiome. Current Opinion in Endocrinology, Diabetes and Obesity, 21(1), 15–21. https://doi.org/10.1097/MED.0000000000000032
- Prinsloo, S., & Lyle, R. (2015). Microbiome, Gut-Brain-Axis, and Implications for Brain Health. NeuroRegulation, 2(4), 158–161. https://doi.org/10.15540/nr.2.4.158
- Quigley, E. (2018). The Gut-Brain Axis and the Microbiome: Clues to Pathophysiology and Opportunities for Novel Management Strategies in Irritable Bowel Syndrome (IBS). Journal of Clinical Medicine, 7(1), 6. https://doi.org/10.3390/jcm7010006
- Quigley, E. M. M. (2016). Overlapping irritable bowel syndrome and inflammatory bowel disease: less to this than meets the eye? Therapeutic Advances in Gastroenterology, 9(2), 199–212. https://doi.org/10.1177/1756283X15621230

Chapter 4: IBD & Nutrition:

- Looijer-van Langen, et al., (2009). Prebiotics in chronic intestinal inflammation. Inflammatory bowel diseases, 15(3), 454–462. https://doi.org/10.1002/ibd.20737
- Hallert C, Kaldma M, Petersson BG. Ispaghula husk may relieve gastrointestinal symptoms in ulcerative colitis in remission. Scand J Gastroenterol 1991;26:747e50
- Fern_andez-Ba~nares F, et al. Randomized clinical trial of Plantago ovata seeds (dietary fiber) as compared with mesalamine in maintaining remission in ulcerative colitis. Spanish Group for the Study of Crohn's Disease and Ulcerative Colitis (GETECCU). Am J Gastroenterol 1999;94:427e33
- Hanai H, Kanauchi O, et al., Germinated barley foodstuff prolongs remission in patients with ulcerative colitis. Int J Mol Med 2004;13:643e7.
- Benjamin JL, Hedin CR, Koutsoumpas A, Ng SC, McCarthy NE, Hart AL, et al. Randomised, double-blind, placebo-controlled trial of fructooligosaccharides in active Crohn's disease. Gut 2011;60:923e9
- Brotherton CS, Taylor AG, et al., A high-fiber diet may improve bowel function and health-related quality of life in patients with Crohn disease. Gastroenterol Nurs 2014;37:206e16
- Chiba M, Tsuji T, Nakane K, Komatsu M. High amount of dietary fiber not harmful but favorable for Crohn disease. Perm J 2015;19:58e61.
- Oliva S, Di Nardo G, et al. Randomised clinical trial: the effectiveness of Lactobacillus reuteri ATCC 55730 rectal enema in children with active distal ulcerative colitis. Aliment Pharmacol Ther 2012;35:327e34
- Miele E, Pascarella F, Giannetti E, Quaglietta L, Baldassano RN, Staiano A. Effect of a probiotic preparation (VSL#3) on induction and maintenance of remission in children with ulcerative colitis. Am J Gastroenterol 2009;104: 437-43

- Fujiya M, Ueno N, Kohgo Y. Probiotic treatments for induction and maintenance of remission in inflammatory bowel diseases: a meta-analysis of randomized controlled trials. Clin J Gastroenterol 2014;7:1e13.
- Kruis W, Fric P, Pokrotnieks J, et al. Maintaining remission of ulcerative colitis with the probiotic Escherichia coli Nissle 1917 is as effective as with standard mesalazine. Gut 2004;53:1617e23.
- Floch MH, Walker WA, et al., Recommendations for probiotic usee2015 update: proceedings and consensus opinion. J Clin Gastroenterol 2015;49(Suppl 1):S69e73.
- Ishikawa H, Matsumoto S, et al. Beneficial effects of probiotic bifidobacterium and galacto-oligosaccharide in patients with ulcerative colitis: a randomized controlled study. Digestion 2011;84:128e33.
- Yoshimatsu Y, Yamada A, Furukawa R, Sono K, Osamura A, Nakamura K, et al. Effectiveness of probiotic therapy for the prevention of relapse in patients with inactive ulcerative colitis. World J Gastroenterol 2015;21:5985e94.
- Meini S, Laureano R, Fani L, Tascini C, Galano A, Antonelli A, et al. Breakthrough Lactobacillus rhamnosus GG bacteremia associated with probiotic use in an adult patient with severe active ulcerative colitis: case report and review of the literature. Infection 2015;43:777e81.
- Vahabnezhad E, Mochon AB, Wozniak LJ, Ziring DA. Lactobacillus bacteremia associated with probiotic use in a pediatric patient with ulcerative colitis. J Clin Gastroenterol 2013;47:437e9
- Gionchetti P, Rizzello F, Morselli C, Poggioli G, et al., High-dose probiotics for the treatment of active pouchitis. Dis Colon Rectum. 2007 Dec;50(12):2075-82; discussion 2082-4. Epub 2007 Oct 13. PMID: 17934776
- Lee JH, Moon G, et al., Effect of a probiotic preparation (VSL#3) in patients with mild to moderate ulcerative colitis. Korean J Gastroenterol. 2012 Aug;60(2):94-101. PMID: 22926120
- Guslandi, M. et al. (2000) Saccharomyces boulardii in Maintenance Treatment of Crohn's Disease. Digestive Diseases & Sciences. Vol 45, 7, 1462 – 1464
- Guslandi M, Giollo P, Testoni PA. A pilot trial of Saccharomyces boulardii in ulcerative colitis. Eur J Gastroenterol Hepatol. 2003 Jun;15(6):697-8. PMID:12840682
- Davani-Davari, D., Negahdaripour, M., et al., (2019). Prebiotics: Definition, Types, Sources, Mechanisms, and Clinical Applications. Foods (Basel, Switzerland), 8(3), 92. https://doi.org/10.3390/foods8030092
- Sunkara, T., Rawla, P., Ofosu, A., & Gaduputi, V. (2018). Fecal microbiota transplant - a new frontier in inflammatory bowel disease. Journal of inflammation research, 11, 321–328. https://doi.org/10.2147/JIR.S176190
- Levy, A. N., & Allegretti, J. R. (2019). Insights into the role of fecal microbiota transplantation for the treatment of inflammatory bowel disease. Therapeutic advances in gastroenterology, 12, 1756284819836893. https://doi.org/10.1177/1756284819836893

- Lopez, J., & Grinspan, A. (2016). Fecal Microbiota Transplantation for Inflammatory Bowel Disease. Gastroenterology & hepatology, 12(6), 374–379.
- van Nood E, Vrieze A, Nieuwdorp M,et al.,(2013). "Duodenal infusion of donor feces for recurrent Clostridium difficile". The New England Journal of Medicine. 368 (5): 407-15
- Paul Moayyedi. Update on Fecal Microbiota Transplantation in Patients With Inflammatory Bowel Disease. Gastroenterology & Hepatology. May 2018 - Volume 14, Issue 5
- Kim, K. O., & Gluck, M. (2019). Fecal Microbiota Transplantation: An Update on Clinical Practice. Clinical endoscopy, 52(2), 137–143. https://doi.org/10.5946/ce.2019.009
- Dimidi, E., Cox, S. R., Rossi, M., & Whelan, K. (2019). Fermented Foods: Definitions and Characteristics, Impact on the Gut Microbiota and Effects on Gastrointestinal Health and Disease. Nutrients, 11(8), 1806. https://doi.org/10.3390/nu11081806
- Melini, F., Melini, V., Luziatelli, F., Ficca, A. G., & Ruzzi, M. (2019). Health-Promoting Components in Fermented Foods: An Up-to-Date Systematic Review. Nutrients, 11(5), 1189. https://doi.org/10.3390/nu11051189
- Bischoff, Stephan C. et al, 2020, ESPEN practical guideline (2020): Clinical Nutrition in inflammatory bowel disease, Clinical Nutrition, Volume 39, Issue 3, 632 – 653
- Fogelholm M, Anderssen S, et al., 2012)., Dietary macronutrients and food consumption as determinants of long-term weight change in adult populations: a systematic literature review. Food Nutr Res. 2012;56:10.3402/fnr.v56i0.19103. doi:10.3402/fnr.v56i0.19103
- British Nutrition Foundation (2018)., [Online], Basics of Nutrition, Available at: https://www.nutrition.org.uk/healthyliving/basics.html
- British Dietetic Association (2018)., [Online] Fat facts: Food Fact Sheet, Available at: https://www.bda.uk.com/uploads/assets 84f584f6-9294-4a5f-8012bf20e7bedd56/Fat-food-fact-sheet.pdf
- Holesh JE, Martin A (2020)., Physiology, Carbohydrates. [Updated 2020 Mar 23]. In: StatPearls [Internet]. Treasure Island (FL): StatPearls Publishing; 2020 Jan-. Available from: https://www.ncbi.nlm.nih.gov/books NBK459280/
- Genetics Home Reference. (2019). What are proteins and what dothey do? Available at: https://ghr.nlm.nih.gov/primer/howgeneswork/protein
- Patterson, E., Wall, R., Fitzgerald, G. F., Ross, R. P., & Stanton, C. (2012). Health implications of high dietary omega-6 polyunsaturated Fatty acids. Journal of nutrition and metabolism, 2012, 539426. https://doi.org/10.1155/2012/539426
- British Nutrition Foundation (2018)., [Online], Energy intake and expenditure, Available at: https://www.nutrition.org.uk/nutritionscience/obesityandweightmanagement/energy-intake-and-expenditure.html?start=1
- Cho HW (2018).,. How Much Caffeine is Too Much for Young Adolescents?. Osong Public Health Res Perspect. 2018;9(6):287-288. doi:10.24171/j.phrp.2018.9.6.01
- Drinkaware (2019)., [Online] The law on alcohol and under 18's, Available at: https://www.drinkaware.co.uk/alcohol-facts/alcohol-and-the-law/the-law-on-alcohol-and-under-18s/

- National Institutes of Health: Office of Dietary Supplements. (2018). Pantothenic Acid. Available at: https://ods.od.nih.gov/factsheets/PantothenicAcid-HealthProfessional/
- National Institutes of Health: Office of Dietary Supplements. (2018). [Online] Biotin, Available at: https://ods.od.nih.gov/factsheets/Biotin-HealthProfessional/
- National Health Service (2020)., [Online], Overview: Vitamins & Minerals, Available at: https://www.nhs.uk/conditions/vitamins-and-minerals/
- Mehanna, H. M., Moledina, J., & Travis, J. (2008). Refeeding syndrome: what it is, and how to prevent and treat it. BMJ (Clinical research ed.), 336(7659), 1495–1498. https://doi.org/10.1136/bmj.a301
- Abbaspour N, Hurrell R, Kelishadi R. Review on iron and its importance for human health. J Res Med Sci. 2014;19(2):164-174.
- British Nutrition Foundation (2018)., [Online], Minerals and trace elements, Available at: https://www.nutrition.org.uk/nutritionscience nutrients-food-and-ingredients/minerals-and-trace-elements.html?limit=1&start=8
- National Institutes of Health: Office of Dietary Supplements. (2018), [Online] Magnesium, Available at: https://ods.od.nih.gov/factsheets/Magnesium-HealthProfessional/
- Strazzullo P, Leclercq C. Sodium. Adv Nutr. 2014;5(2):188-190. Published 2014 Mar 1. doi:10.3945/an.113.005215
- Sahay M, Sahay R. Hyponatremia: A practical approach. Indian J Endocrinol Metab. 2014;18(6):760-771. doi:10.4103/2230-8210.141320
- BMJ Best Practice (2020). Assessment of anaemia. [Online] https://bestpractice.bmj.com/topics/en-gb/93
- Larussa, T., Suraci, E., Marasco, R., Imeneo, M., Abenavoli, L., & Luzza, F. (2019). Self-Prescribed Dietary Restrictions are Common in Inflammatory Bowel Disease Patients and Are Associated with Low Bone Mineralization. Medicina (Kaunas, Lithuania), 55(8), 507. https://doi.org/10.3390/medicina55080507
- Swanson, G. R., Sedghi, S., Farhadi, A., & Keshavarzian, A. (2010). Pattern of alcohol consumption and its effect on gastrointestinal symptoms in inflammatory bowel disease. Alcohol (Fayetteville, N.Y.), 44(3), 223–228. https://doi.org/10.1016/j.alcohol.2009.10.019
- Mantzouranis, G., Fafliora, E., et al., 2018). Alcohol and narcotics use in inflammatory bowel disease. Annals of gastroenterology, 31(6), 649–658. https://doi.org/10.20524/aog.2018.0302
- Cannon, A. R., Kuprys, P. V., et al., (2018). Alcohol enhances symptoms and propensity for infection in inflammatory bowel disease patients and a murine model of DSS-induced colitis. Journal of leukocyte biology, 104(3), 543–555. https://doi.org/10.1002/JLB.4MA1217-506R
- Bishehsari, F., Magno, E., Swanson, G., Desai, V., Voigt, R. M., Forsyth, C. B., & Keshavarzian, A. (2017). Alcohol and Gut-Derived Inflammation. Alcohol research: current reviews, 38(2), 163–171.
- Fawehinmi TO, Ilomäki J, Voutilainen S, Kauhanen J (2012)., Alcohol consumption and dietary patterns: the FinDrink study. PLoS One. 2012;7(6):e38607. doi:10.1371/journal.pone.0038607

- Brown AC, Rampertab SD, Mullin GE. Existing dietary guidelines for Crohn's disease and ulcerative colitis. Expert Rev Gastroenterol Hepatol. 2011 Jun;5(3):411-25. doi: 10.1586/egh.11.29. PMID: 21651358
- Rapuri PB, Gallagher JC, Kinyamu HK, Ryschon KL. Caffeine intake increases the rate of bone loss in elderly women and interacts with vitamin D receptor genotypes. Am J Clin Nutr. 2001 Nov;74(5):694-700. PMID: 11684540
- Boekema PJ, Samsom M, van Berge Henegouwen GP, Smout AJ. Coffee and gastrointestinal function: facts and fiction. A review. Scand J Gastroenterol Suppl. 1999;230:35-9. PMID: 10499460

Chapter 5: IBD Diets, Stomas & Nutritional Therapy

- Rizzello, F., Spisni, E., Giovanardi, E., Imbesi, V., Salice, M., Alvisi, P., Valerii, M. C., & Gionchetti, P. (2019). Implications of the Westernized Diet in the Onset and Progression of IBD. Nutrients, 11(5), 1033. https://doi.org/10.3390/nu11051033
- Pigneur, B., & Ruemmele, F. M. (2019). Nutritional interventions for the treatment of IBD: current evidence and controversies. Therapeutic advances in gastroenterology, 12, 1756284819890534. https://doi.org/10.1177/1756284819890534
- Tuck, C. J., Biesiekierski, J et al., (2019). Food Intolerances. Nutrients, 11(7), 1684. https://doi.org/10.3390/nu11071684
- Lopez CM, Yarrarapu SNS, Mendez MD. Food Allergies. [Updated 2020 Sep 11]. In: StatPearls [Internet]. Treasure Island (FL): StatPearls Publishing; 2020 Jan-. Available from: https://www.ncbi.nlm.nih.gov/books NBK482187/
- Reddavide, R., Rotolo, O et al., (2018). The role of diet in the prevention and treatment of Inflammatory Bowel Diseases. Acta biomedica : Atenei Parmensis, 89(9-S), 60–75. https://doi.org/10.23750/abm.v89i9-S.7952
- Green, N., Miller, T., Suskind, D., & Lee, D. (2019). A Review of Dietary Therapy for IBD and a Vision for the Future. Nutrients, 11(5), 947. https://doi.org/10.3390/nu11050947
- Kakodkar, Samir et al (2015), The Specific Carbohydrate Diet for Inflammatory Bowel Disease: A Case Series Journal of the Academy of Nutrition and Dietetics, Volume 115, Issue 8, 1226 - 1232
- Mentella, M. C., Scaldaferri, F., Pizzoferrato, M., Gasbarrini, A., & Miggiano, G. (2020). Nutrition, IBD and Gut Microbiota: A Review. Nutrients, 12(4), 944. https://doi.org/10.3390/nu12040944
- Gibson, P. R. (2017) Use of the low-FODMAP diet in inflammatory bowel disease. Journal of Gastroenterology and Hepatology, 32: 40–42. doi: 10.1111/jgh.13695.
- Pedersen, N., Ankersen, D. V., Felding, M., Wachmann, H., Végh, Z., Molzen, L., Burisch, J., Andersen, J. R., & Munkholm, P. (2017). Low-FODMAP diet reduces irritable bowel symptoms in patients with inflammatory bowel disease. World journal of gastroenterology, 23(18), 3356–3366. https://doi.org/10.3748/wjg.v23.i18.3356
- Donnellan, C. F., Yann, L. H., & Lal, S. (2013). Nutritional management of Crohn's disease. Therapeutic advances in gastroenterology, 6(3), 231–242. https://doi.org/10.1177/1756283X13477715
- Kakodkar, S., & Mutlu, E. A. (2017). Diet as a Therapeutic Option for Adult Inflammatory Bowel Disease. Gastroenterology clinics of North America, 46(4), 745–767. https://doi.org/10.1016/j.gtc.2017.08.016

- Festen EA, Goyette P et al, A meta-analysis of genome-wide association scans identifies IL18RAP, PTPN2, TAGAP, and PUS10 as shared risk loci for Crohn's disease and celiac disease. PLoS Genet. 2011 Jan 27;7(1):e1001283. doi: 10.1371/journal.pgen.1001283

- Alberto Rubio-Tapia, Robert A. Kyle et al., (2009), Increased Prevalence and Mortality in Undiagnosed Celiac Disease. Gastroenterology. 2009 Jul;137(1):88-93. doi: 10.1053/j.gastro.2009.03.059. Epub 2009 Apr 10.

- Haskey, N., & Gibson, D. L. (2017). An Examination of Diet for the Maintenance of Remission in Inflammatory Bowel Disease. Nutrients, 9(3), 259. https://doi.org/10.3390/nu9030259

- Knight-Sepulveda, K., Kais, S., Santaolalla, R., & Abreu, M. T. (2015). Diet and Inflammatory Bowel Disease. Gastroenterology & hepatology, 11(8), 511–520

- Castro, F., & de Souza, H. (2019). Dietary Composition and Effects in Inflammatory Bowel Disease. Nutrients, 11(6), 1398. https://doi.org/10.3390/nu11061398

- Narula, N., Dhillon, A., Zhang, D., Sherlock, M. E., Tondeur, M., & Zachos, M. (2018). Enteral nutritional therapy for induction of remission in Crohn's disease. The Cochrane database of systematic reviews, 4(4), CD000542. https://doi.org/10.1002 14651858.CD000542.pub3

- Rolandsdotter, H., Jönsson-Videsäter, K., L Fagerberg, U., Finkel, Y., & Eberhardson, M. (2019). Exclusive Enteral Nutrition: Clinical Effects and Changes in Mucosal Cytokine Profile in Pediatric New Inflammatory Bowel Disease. Nutrients, 11(2), 414. https://doi.org/10.3390/nu11020414

- Hansen, T., & Duerksen, D. R. (2018). Enteral Nutrition in the Management of Pediatric and Adult Crohn's Disease. Nutrients, 10(5), 537. https://doi.org/10.3390/nu10050537

- Andoh A, Inoue R, Kawada Y, et al. Elemental diet induces alterations of the gut microbial community in mice. Journal of Clinical Biochemistry and Nutrition. 2019 Sep;65(2):118-124. DOI: 10.3164/jcbn.19-8.

- Chiba, M., Ishii, H., & Komatsu, M. (2019). Recommendation of plant-based diets for inflammatory bowel disease. Translational pediatrics, 8(1), 23–27. https://doi.org/10.21037/tp.2018.12.02

- Comeche, J. M., Comino, I, et al., (2019). Parenteral Nutrition in Patients with Inflammatory Bowel Disease Systematic Review, Meta-Analysis and Meta-Regression. Nutrients, 11(12), 2865. https://doi.org/10.3390/nu11122865

- Semrad C. E. (2012). Use of parenteral nutrition in patients with inflammatory bowel disease. Gastroenterology & hepatology, 8(6), 393–395.

- Schulz, R. J., Bischoff, S. C., et al., (2009). Gastroenterology - Guidelines on Parenteral Nutrition, Chapter 15. German medical science: GMS e-journal, 7, Doc13. https://doi.org/10.3205/000072

- Ambe, P. C., Kurz, N. R., Nitschke, C., Odeh, S. F., Möslein, G., & Zirngibl, H. (2018). Intestinal Ostomy. Deutsches Arzteblatt international, 115(11), 182–187. https://doi.org/10.3238/arztebl.2018.0182

- United Ostomy Association of America, Eating with an Ostomy, [Online], Available at: https://www.ostomy.org/wp-content/uploads/2020/07/Eating_with_an_Os tomy_2020-07.pdf

Chapter 6: Common IBD Issues

- Dossett, M. L., Cohen, E. M., & Cohen, J. (2017). Integrative Medicine for Gastrointestinal Disease. Primary care, 44(2), 265–280. https://doi.org/10.1016/j.pop.2017.02.002
- Klenzak, S., Danelisen, I., et al., (2018). Management of gastroesophageal reflux disease: Patient and physician communication challenges and shared decision making. World journal of clinical cases, 6(15), 892–900. https://doi.org/10.12998/wjcc.v6.i15.892
- Antunes C, Aleem A, Curtis SA. Gastroesophageal Reflux Disease. [Updated 2020 Jul 8]. In: StatPearls [Internet]. Treasure Island (FL): StatPearls Publishing; 2020 Jan-. Available from: https://www.ncbi.nlm.nih.gov/books/NBK44 1938/
- Christine Norton, Lesley B. Dibley, Paul Bassett, Faecal incontinence in inflammatory bowel disease: Associations and effect on quality of life, Journal of Crohn's and Colitis, Volume 7, Issue 8, September 2013, Pages e302–e311, https://doi.org/10.1016/j.crohns.2012.11.00 4
- Barros, L. L., Farias, A. Q., & Rezaie, A. (2019). Gastrointestinal motility and absorptive disorders in patients with inflammatory bowel diseases: Prevalence, diagnosis and treatment. World journal of gastroenterology, 25(31), 4414–4426. https://doi.org/10.3748/wjg.v25.i31.4414
- Saldana Ruiz, N., & Kaiser, A. M. (2017). Fecal incontinence - Challenges and solutions. World journal of gastroenterology, 23(1), 11–24. https://doi.org/10.3748/wjg.v23.i1.11
- Nemeth V, Pfleghaar N. Diarrhea. [Updated 2020 Jul 19]. In: StatPearls [Internet]. Treasure Island (FL): StatPearls Publishing; 2020 Jan-. Available from: https://www.ncbi.nlm.nih.gov/books/NBK44 8082/
- Anbazhagan, A. N., Priyamvada, S., Alrefai, W. A., & Dudeja, P. K. (2018). Pathophysiology of IBD associated diarrhea. Tissue barriers, 6(2), e1463897. https://doi.org/10.1080/21688370.2018.1463 897
- Akbar, A., Yiangou, Y., Facer, P., Walters, J. R. F., Anand, P., & Ghosh, S. (2008). Increased capsaicin receptor TRPV1-expressing sensory fibres in irritable bowel syndrome and their correlation with abdominal pain. Gut, 57, 923–929. https://doi.org/10.1136/gut.2007.138982
- MacDermott, R. P. (2007). Treatment of irritable bowel syndrome in outpatients with inflammatory bowel disease using a food and beverage intolerance, food and beverage avoidance diet. Inflammatory Bowel Diseases, 13(1), 91–96. https://doi.org/10.1002/ibd.20048
- Lacy, B. E., Gabbard, S. L., & Crowell, M. D. (2011). Pathophysiology, evaluation, and treatment of bloating: hope, hype, or hot air?. Gastroenterology & hepatology, 7(11), 729–739.
- Seo, A. Y., Kim, N., & Oh, D. H. (2013). Abdominal bloating: pathophysiology and treatment. Journal of neurogastroenterology and motility, 19(4), 433–453. https://doi.org/10.5056/jnm.2013.19.4.433
- Bordoni, B., & Morabito, B. (2018). Symptomatology Correlations Between the Diaphragm and Irritable Bowel Syndrome. Cureus, 10(7), e3036. https://doi.org/10.7759/cureus.3036

- Sorathia SJ, Rivas JM. Small Intestinal Bacterial Overgrowth. [Updated 2020 Jun 29]. In: StatPearls [Internet]. Treasure Island (FL): StatPearls Publishing; 2020 Jan-. Available from: https://www.ncbi.nlm.nih.gov/books NBK546634/
- Mawer S, Alhawaj AF. Physiology, Defecation. [Updated 2020 Sep 13]. In: StatPearls [Internet]. Treasure Island (FL): StatPearls Publishing; 2020 Jan-. Available from: https://www.ncbi.nlm.nih.gov/books NBK539732/
- Andrews, C. N., & Storr, M. (2011). The pathophysiology of chronic constipation. Canadian journal of gastroenterology = Journal canadien de gastroenterologie, 25 Suppl B(Suppl B), 16B–21B.
- Modi, R. M., Hinton, A., Pinkhas, D., Groce, R., Meyer, M. M., Balasubramanian, G., Levine, E., & Stanich, P. P. (2019). Implementation of a Defecation Posture Modification Device: Impact on Bowel Movement Patterns in Healthy Subjects. Journal of clinical gastroenterology, 53(3), 216–219. https://doi.org/10.1097/MCG.000000000000 1143
- Diaz S, Bittar K, Mendez MD. Constipation. [Updated 2020 Jul 26]. In: StatPearls [Internet]. Treasure Island (FL): StatPearls Publishing; 2020 Jan-. Available from: https://www.ncbi.nlm.nih.gov/books NBK513291/

INDEX

N

Nausea (69,73,78)

O

Obesity (27, 72)
Oxalate (26,57)

P

Parenteral Nutrition (40,56,60,83,84)
Pathogenesis (28)
Percutaneous Abscess Drainage (85)
Perianal Fistula (85,93,)
Peristalsis (19,22,96)
Prebiotics (63, 64, 77)
Probiotics (63, 64, 78)

R

RAIR (23)
Rectovaginal Fistula (85)
Refeeding Syndrome (56,60)

S

Selenosis (60)
Sepsis (86)
Seton (85)
Stenosis (87)
Stoma (41,79, 81)
Stricture (35, 64, 65, 86, 87)
Symbiosis (79)

T

Tenesmus (93)
Toxic Megacolon (86)
Transferrin (37)
Trigger Food (70, 73-75, 77, 96)

U

Ulcerative Colitis (17, 22, 25, 30-33, 45, 50, 54, 57-58, 63-64, 67, 71, 86)
Ultrasound (35, 39)

V

Vegan (79)
Vegetarian (64,79,)
Vitamins (53-57)

W

Western Diet (9, 27, 72, 74)

X

Xenobiotic (26)
Xerophthalmia (54)
X-ray (12,35,39,83)

Acknowledgements

I want to start off by thanking my parents. This book is dedicated to you both and I feel no matter what I do for you I will never ever be able to repay you for always being there for me. There are no words that can convey my gratitude and love for you both. I would also like to thank my siblings for their constant support and input into this book from the art work, cover design and recipes.

I would also like to thank my close friends who have always been so supportive and understanding when it came to telling them about my crohn's disease and helping me find the humour in my condition.

Lastly, and by no means least, I want to thank all my followers on my social media. I never reall took notice of the numbers but your support of my pages through either liking, commenting or sharing my posts and YouTube videos means alot. Especially as it helps to raise awareness of IBD and de-stigmatise the disease. Thank you for following my journey and inspiring me to want to contirbute to the chronic illness community.